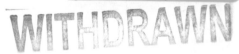

The Malpractice Cure

How to Avoid the Legal Mistakes That Doctors Make

by Edward D. McCarthy

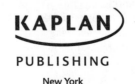

KAPLAN

PUBLISHING

New York

This publication is designed to provide accurate and authoritative information in regard to the subject matter covered. It is sold with the understanding that the publisher is not engaged in rendering legal, accounting, or other professional service. If legal advice or other expert assistance is required, the services of a competent professional should be sought.

Published by Kaplan Publishing, a division of Kaplan, Inc.
1 Liberty Plaza, 24th Floor
New York, NY 10006

Printed in the United States of America

10 9 8 7 6 5 4 3 2 1

Library of Congress Cataloging-in-Publication Data

McCarthy, Edward D., 1939-
    The malpractice cure : how to avoid the legal mistakes that doctors make / Edward McCarthy.
        p. cm.
    ISBN-13: 978-1-4277-9959-3 (pbk.)
    ISBN-10: 1-4277-9959-8 (pbk.)
    1. Physicians—Malpractice—United States. I. Title.
    KF2905.3.M354 2009
    347.7304'121—dc22

                                        2009000513

Table of Contents

Chapter 3
Hospital Settings 77

Chapter 4
Adverse Events 161

Chapter 5
Conclusion 199

Glossary

Abandonment—A one-way termination of the physician-patient relationship by the physician, without the patient's consent, when the patient reasonably requires medical attention and the physician has not made arrangements for appropriate follow-up

Administrator—Someone appointed by family court to handle the estate of a deceased person

Admissibility—Evidence that may be considered in a legal proceeding

Affidavit—A sworn statement, usually in writing

Allegation—A factual statement that a party claims to be able to prove

Answer—The doctor's written response to a complaint

Appeal—The procedural description of what happens when a decision of a lower court is brought to a higher court for review

Burden of proof—The requirement or duty of affirmatively proving some fact or facts in dispute on an issue raised between the parties

Causation—A connection between the alleged acts of the defendant and the injury suffered by the plaintiff, usually requiring proof that the plaintiff's harm or injury resulted proximately from the physician's negligence

Complaint—The first written claim filed in court by a plaintiff in a civil lawsuit, generally designed merely to give the defendant notice of the alleged facts, which constitute the claim.

Consent—A voluntary act by which one person agrees to another to allow another person to do something

Contributory or comparative negligence—A possible defense to a malpractice case, asserting that the patient's negligence may have contributed to the patient's own injury, even though the physican may have also been responsible

Damages—Monetary amounts received through a judicial order as a result of a trial or claim

Decedent—A dead person, ordinarily the injured person, who would have been described as the plaintiff if still living

Defendant—The person against whom a civil claim is brought

Deposition—The testimony of a witness or a party taken before trial consisting of an oral, sworn, out-of-court statement. In medical malpractice cases, both sides of the case are subjected to oral depositions, generally at the office of the opposing counsel. This is done under oath. Generally, the deposition is part of the discovery process, and your lawyer may choose not to ask you any questions at the time of the oral deposition, preferring to reserve questions until the time of trial.

Discovery—Pretrial actions of the parties to a case to attempt to learn of all potential evidence known by the

opposing party or witnesses and to minimize surprises
at the time of trial

Duty—Broadly, the obligation of the physician to treat a
patient according to the required standard of care

Evidence—Broadly, the testimony of witnesses, records, documents, exhibits, objects, and photographs, all of which
may be offered to support the claim of either party

Executor—The person who is appointed under the will of a
deceased person (The executor should not be confused
with administrator, who is appointed by the family court
when a person does not leave a will. Essentially, they
perform the same function.)

Expert witness—An individual with special training, knowledge, skill, or experience in an area pertinent to the
case, which would be beyond the average knowledge of
a juror or lay person, who is allowed to offer opinion
testimony in court

Fiduciary—A person, such as a guardian, conservator, administrator, executor, etc., who is in a position of confidence
or trust and is acting on behalf of another person

Foreseeability—The reasonable expectation that some
injury may happen as a result of something that the
physicial does or fails to do

Immunity—A legal protection given to some individuals that
may protect them from personal liability (For example,
charitable hospitals generally have a limited immunity
up to a certain dollar amount, and governmental employees, such as house officers and physicians in governmental hospitals, have personal immunity.)

Informed consent—The voluntary assent by a patient to accept treatment based upon what the patient knows about the plan and/or course of the proposed treatment, the alternative treatments, or the choice of no treatment at all

Injury—The damage or harm to a patient caused by the physician's breech of duty toward that patient

Interrogatory—Written questions between the parties to a lawsuit as part of discovery

Jury—A certain number of persons, variable from state to state, who are selected according to the law and procedure of the particular state and are sworn to determine the issues before them, with a judge presiding over the case who instructs them on the law in a particular jurisdiction

Litigation—In the broadest of terms, the process of resolution of a dispute in a court of law or by a mediator or arbitrator to determine the factual and legal rights and duties between the parties to a lawsuit

Malice—A wrongful act, more than simple negligence, with an intent to cause an injury to a person implied

Malpractice—So-called professional or medical negligence, meaning a failure to meet a professional standard of care resulting in injury to another

Motion—A written document sent to a court requesting that a judge make an order or ruling, which may be pertinent to the lawsuit

Negligence—As applied to medical malpractice cases, the failure of a physician to act as a reasonable physician, or the failure to comply with the standard of care of an average qualified physician in that setting or in that specialty

Opinion evidence—Evidence generally given by experts based on their special training or background

Pain and suffering—Elements of damages that allow recovery for the mental or physical pain or injuries suffered by a claimant as a result of the injury that is the subject of their claim

Plaintiff—The person who files or begins a civil lawsuit looking for compensation, generally in medical malpractice cases the defendant's patient or former patient

Pleadings—The documents that the parties file back and forth in a case to try to narrow the issues in the case

Proximate cause—A requirement that a plaintiff show in a medical malpractice case that an alleged negligent act proximately caused, or was a substantial contributing factor in causing, the injury in question

Release—A document signed by a person, usually the plaintiff in the case, waiving or giving up a right or claim against a defendant, generally based upon a payment of money

Settlement—The agreement between the parties to a lawsuit that resolves their claim

Statute of limitations—Legal statutes, generally enacted by state legislatures, that specify the interval between something happening and the time when a person may file a lawsuit (If a party fails to bring a lawsuit generally within those time limits, the case may be dismissed.)

Subpoena—A court order requiring a person to appear to give testimony or to produce records

Summons—Generally the first paper, together with the complaint, served upon a defendant in a civil claim; calls for the filing of an answer

Tort—The legal term for a civil wrong, meaning that the allegation is not criminal but alleges that someone has violated a duty to another

Verdict—A binding decision regarding all manners of fact submitted to a jury or fact finder, who may be a judge, arbitrator, or mediator

Vicarious liability—Secondary liability that may be imposed upon the physician because of the actions of someone who is employed by the physician or over whom the physician exercises a certain amount of control, such as an office secretary, nurse, or—in a hospital setting—even a house officer

Introduction

THIS HANDBOOK IS MEANT to be a useful guide for practicing healthcare providers, including physicians, dentists, nurse practitioners, physicians' assistants, nurse midwives, nurses, technicians, and other staff. While numerous publications advise the provider about what to do if a claim is actually made against them, little, if anything, has been written with respect to practical suggestions for avoiding the unpleasant process altogether. While the suggestions in this book are based on four decades of experience in representing healthcare providers, they are not meant as legal advice or as a substitute for advice from your own attorney, a hospital attorney, and/or risk manager of a health facility. When in doubt, always speak with that person. This book is meant to prevent or at least minimize the likelihood of having to endure a lawsuit that can drag on for years, leaving a bitter aftertaste even when the result has been favorable to you.

My practice in the late 1960s and early 1970s gradually shifted to the medical legal area. As assistant city solicitor of the City of Cambridge, Massachusetts, from 1964 to 1971 and city solicitor from 1971 to 1976, I also served as counsel to the Cambridge Hospital, dealing with all of its legal matters, including litigation. In about 1975, with the explosion of so-called medical malpractice lawsuits, I began to practice exclusively in the medical legal area. I became counsel for Cambridge Hospital, which later separated from the City of Cambridge to form the Cambridge Public Health Commission, consisting of the Cambridge Hospital, Somerville Hospital, and the Whidden Hospital in Everett, Massachusetts, as well as a number of freestanding clinics. These facilities all continued their long-standing affiliation with Harvard University Medical School.

At the same time, other members of my firm and I acted as defense lawyers in medical claims for the Risk Management Foundation of the Harvard Medical Institutions, ProMutual Group (formerly the Massachusetts Joint Underwriting Association), Tufts University Medical Center, the Boston Medical Center (affiliated with Boston University Medical School), and University of Massachusetts Medical Center, as well as a number of other specialized and smaller carriers.

In the early 1990s, I had the great enjoyment of teaching Health and Hospital Law at the New England School of Law in Boston; I eventually left because of a full trial schedule. In 2003, I left the position of general counsel of the Cambridge Public Health Commission and, since that time, continue actively in the defense of medical malpractice claims for the various insurers previously mentioned.

Throughout the years, I've had the pleasure and privilege of representing many of the most honorable, dedicated professional men and women in the medical field. This book, in a small way, is meant to help them and others to come after them to avoid unpleasant conflicts between patient and provider, which end up being resolved in a forum and under terms totally foreign to you as providers.

The realities of the marketplace have imposed unreasonable demands on the time of the provider, adversely affecting the patient relationship and setting the stage for lawsuits. Over the years, my colleagues and I have seen many cases that could have been avoided by things as simple as more legible records, more courteous staff, better personal relations with the patient, better systems management, better overall information collection, and better informing of the patient. None of these factors reflects upon the state of medical knowledge of the provider; rather, they influence the perception of the patient, which affects the overall tone of the relationship. System errors can be diligently watched out for and corrected, and things as simple as legibility of records can likewise be corrected with minimal effort.

If you find yourself in a situation where you are the subject of a claim, there are some materials in the latter part of the book to head you in the right direction. This is not meant to be a scholarly work but a book written in a conversational tone in which I share experiences that I feel can be helpful to you.

Chapter 1

Claims Against Healthcare Providers

LEGAL PRINCIPLES

The legal principles are essentially the same for all health-care providers, regardless of the level of care they are rendering or their specialties. For ease of discussion, I will refer to healthcare providers as "physicians" or "doctors," with the understanding that I am being inclusive of all health-care providers.

Standard of Care

For a patient to recover in a medical negligence or so-called medical malpractice case against a physician, the patient must do three things:

1. *Prove that the physician did not act as a reasonably prudent doctor.* This principle is worded differently from state to state but is sometimes referred to as "a burden" that the patient has to prove that the physician deviated from the "standard of care." *Standard of care* means that degree of care exercised by the average qualified provider given the circumstances. For example, the standard of care for a specialist would be the standard of the average qualified specialist.
2. *Prove that, if indeed there was a departure from the standard of care, the departure caused an injury or damage.*
3. *Prove damages.*

Burden of Proof

Burden of proof means that the patient needs to convince a fact finder, whether it be a jury, a judge, or an arbitrator, that the patient's claim is more probably true than not. Sometimes, this probability is given an arithmetic value, and judges will tell a jury that if they feel that this case is 50/50, then the patient (usually referred to as the plaintiff) has not proved the case, but if they find that the evidence tips in favor of the plaintiff, then the plaintiff has met the burden of proof.

Loss of Chance

This doctrine, which has been adopted by about 20 states and the District of Columbia, recognizes the right of a plaintiff patient to recover for a loss of chance alone, even though the physician may not be liable for the ultimate harm or injury. This is a very complicated theory to understand and will create interesting situations for juries.

This doctrine was adopted most recently in Massachusetts; the case, *Matsuyama v. Birnbaum,* was decided on July 23, 2008. The patient alleged that the doctor should have diagnosed his gastric cancer between 1995 and his eventual diagnosis in May 1999. The jury found that the patient was suffering from stage II adenocarcinoma at the time of the doctor's initial negligence and, based upon the statistical evidence of the experts, had a 37.5 percent chance of survival at that time. This, of course, means that there was a 62.5 percent chance that the underlying disease would cause the patient's death. The Massachusetts Supreme Court, as have the courts in the other states where the doctrine of loss of chance has been adopted, recognized that the loss of chance is something that can be compensated on its own. In this case, it awarded $875,000 as "full" wrongful death damages, multiplied that amount by the survival rate of 0.375, and entered a judgment in the sum of $328,125.

The jury also found that the doctor's negligence was a "substantial contributing factor" to the death. Part of the justification for this decision was the feeling of the court that much treatment today is aimed at extending life, even for brief periods, and improving the quality of life without curing the underlying condition. The Court gave an example: If a jury found that full wrongful death damages were $600,000, but the patient had a 45 percent chance of survival prior to the claimed medical negligence and a 15 percent chance due to the negligence, then the patient's survival was reduced by 30 percent, and the damages would be $600,000 multiplied by 0.30, or $180,000.

In another case decided on the same day, *Renzi v. Paredes,* Massachusetts found that a plaintiff in a breast cancer case was entitled to loss of chance damages, even though the jury found that neither of the two physicians caused the death. In other words, no wrongful death damages were awarded, but separate damages were awarded for the "loss of chance" to survive. I'm certain that this is confusing to a healthcare provider, as it is confusing to lawyers in the field. These cases illustrate some of the potential liability dangers that lurk and reinforce the need for diligence in avoiding claims.

These legal rulings are not necessarily reflective of the true state of medicine on issues of loss of chance and causation. The average layperson believes what he has heard for years—that early detection of cancer equals a greater chance of survival. However, this understanding may not necessarily have a good scientific basis.

Cancers are generally thought to be clinically detectable when they are about 1 centimeter in size and contain about 1 billion cancer cells. How can detection be "early" when the cancer has grown to 80 percent of its eventual, fatal size? Recent studies of human genetics and the biology of some stage I tumors have shown that different patients with stage I cancer may have low, moderate, or high risk of recurrence or metastasis. Therefore, staging isn't a truly accurate predictor of survivability. Staging was designed to assist in treatment of patients, not to be the basis of legal claims. Until the legal theory catches up with medicine, it may be advisable not to paint rosy pictures for patients based on staging. I have had doctors tell me, "I cured a patient's colon cancer today," when, in reality, they really didn't know. Patients need to have hope, but you need to be a bit conservative in making blanket statements about the future.

Duty to Warn

Another recent case, also in Massachusetts, recognized liability against a physician whose alleged failure to warn a patient about the risks of driving while taking prescription medications allegedly resulted in an automobile accident and injuries to third parties, who were permitted to recover damages directly against the physician. *Coombes v. Florio* was decided on December 10, 2007. Of the six judges participating in the decision, three found that the liability of the doctor extended to third parties who were not in a patient relationship with the doctor, one judge agreed in part, and two judges dissented or disagreed.

Part of the process of learning to avoid claims is being aware of the nature of some of the claims that can be made. In *Coombes,* a 10-year-old boy was killed by an automobile driven by a patient of the defendant doctor. The patient was 75 years old and had a number of serious medical conditions, including asbestosis, chronic bronchitis, emphysema, high blood pressure, and metastatic lung cancer that had spread to his lymph nodes. The physician was the primary care physician and was responsible for all of this older patient's medications. The doctor had earlier warned the patient that it would not be safe to drive during his cancer treatment, and the patient said that he complied and did not drive until the conclusion of those treatments, at which time the doctor advised him that he could safely resume driving. At the time of the accident, the patient was taking oxycodone, zaroxolyn, prednisone, flomax, potassium, paxil, oxazepam, and furosemide. The potential side effects of the drugs included drowsiness, dizziness, light-headedness, fainting, altered consciousness, and sedation. The family had an expert who would testify that the drugs in combination could cause additive side effects, which could be more severe than the side effects when the drugs were used separately.

The patient had reported no side effects and reported no difficulty with driving. Neither was there anything in the record of a warning to the patient of any potential side effects. You probably could understand the validity of a claim by the *patient* that the physician failed to adequately warn him of the potential side effects of the medication. However, this case went farther, allowing a *third party*, the family of this 10-year-old, to recover directly against the doctor for negligence in failing to warn his patient. The court found that the doctor was negligent in prescribing the medication without warning of the potential side effects and that that duty extended to this young boy, because the boy's injury and death was a foreseeable consequence of the negligence.

In the dissenting opinion, Judge Cordy disagreed with the findings, asking: "Is the doctor to tell the patient whenever a medication is prescribed that might in some circumstance cause drowsiness or fainting, 'Do not drive. Do not hold your grandchild. Do not carry grocery bags to your car. In fact, do not do anything that involves interacting with another person?'"

This claim might have been prevented by careful documentation of a discussion with the patient of the risks involved with taking all of these medications, taking into account the patient's overall medical condition, and a discussion of whether it was safe for him to operate a motor vehicle. If the physician had documented that the warnings indeed were given to the patient, the liability would not have extended to people outside of the physician-patient relationship. This rule is generally recognized in Hawaii, Maine, South Carolina, and Tennessee.

I should point out that, as of this date, Illinois and Kansas have declined to impose such a duty to third parties in similar circumstances. In Pennsylvania, however, an older case holds that a physician had a duty to a man, whom the doctor had never met, who contracted hepatitis from a female patient to whom the doctor allegedly gave erroneous advice regarding the communicable nature of the disease. In a pending case in the Massachusetts Supreme Judicial Court, *Leavitt v. Brockton Hospital*, the issue is "whether a hospital and its employees, who in disregard of accepted practices, discharged a sedated patient post colonoscopy without an adult escort, owed a duty of care to a police officer who was injured in an automobile accident while en route to aid the impaired patient who had been fatally injured in a separate pedestrian-automobile accident while walking home alone." This case was filed in a trial court and dismissed by a judge, and that ruling is the subject of appeal.

Such cases occur all over the country. Forewarned is forearmed. Duty to warn is a developing area of the law, and you need to be aware of it.

As a matter of fact, as this book is going to press, I just read a case, decided on November 25, 2008, in which a limousine driver was held liable for dropping off a drunken passenger (who had the foresight to attend a bachelor party with a limousine driver) who then got into his own automobile and had an accident resulting in a fatality. This is a real stretch of liability from the precedent of many years. It does not bode well for duty to warn cases relative to healthcare providers. Be forewarned.

Causation and Damages

The claimant also has to prove the element of causation. In other words, the claimant has the burden of proving that, even if you departed from the standard of care, that departure actually caused some injury or damage. For example, if you had been following a patient's prostate-specific antigen (PSA) levels at annual physicals and for some reason forgot to order the test in a particular year, it might be argued that not ordering it was a departure from the standard of care. However, if the patient had a PSA level drawn a year later and it was in keeping with prior PSA levels, then there obviously would have been no injury caused to the patient. In one case, I saw a jury find that an emergency room doctor was negligent in failing to make arrangements for a stroke patient to consult with a neurologist and possibly receive treatment with tissue plasminogen activator (tPA). The timing of the stroke was in dispute, and the jury found that that conduct did not cause the stroke or a worsening of the stroke or lessen the chance of recovery, because the patient was outside the three-hour treatment window.

To establish the standard of care, causation, and damages, the patient ordinarily has to present expert testimony to the fact finder. In some cases, however, a fact finder might infer that the provider was negligent merely because the circumstances of the case are such that they would not have happened unless the provider had been negligent. This is known as *res ipsa loquitur,* or "the thing or matter speaks for itself." The patient would have to also show that whatever caused the injury was under the care and management of the provider involved and that the provider possessed better knowledge and had more information about the cause of the injury. The doctrine has been applied in cases of retained sponges, towels, and instruments during surgery. In a 2000 case where the patient had a total right knee replacement and awoke with pain in her right hand, right arm, and right shoulder, the Missouri Court of Appeals found that this kind of injury would not occur without negligence.

The *res ipsa loquitur* doctrine creates an inference of negligence. In these cases, the defendant must introduce evidence to show that there wasn't any negligence on the part of the provider. The doctrine has been applied to cases involving a burn to the calf following surgery to the foot, a nerve injury to the arm following surgery to the spine, injury to the neck during proctoscopic examination, and similar types of cases, such as a dentist dropping an instrument that ended up in the patient's stomach.

Expert reports and/or testimony in a medical negligence case are not necessarily what you would expect to hear at a professional meeting. The standard of care at a trial will be determined by the fact finder based on the credibility, believability, and expertise of the experts for both sides. The usual case involves a plaintiff's having an expert say one thing and the defendant's having an expert say another thing and then a jury's making a determination. This process, in and of itself, is a good reason to make efforts to stay clear of this kind of setting.

There are hundreds of examples, but one that stands out in my mind is the typical cerebral palsy case. For decades, physicians have been involved in defending these very high damage cases. A jury is presented with an incredibly sympathetic young child, who may be confined to a wheelchair for the rest of her life because of an incident claimed by the plaintiff to have occurred during the labor and delivery process. Most of the good medical evidence over the years shows that science really does not know the cause of cerebral palsy alleged to have occurred as part of the labor and delivery process; and in spite of various monitoring improvements, the rate of cerebral palsy has not decreased. Nonetheless, in some of these exceedingly sympathetic cases, an expert for the plaintiff may carry the day through the sympathy factor. Some of these experts travel around the country testifying in case after case, really as a full-time occupation, and may do very little in the practice of medicine. Even when this information is brought out at a trial, again the jury's sympathies tend to carry the day.

Physicians always ask, "How can this case possibly go forward? No self-respecting expert would say something like that." Regrettably, we show them these expert reports, and the case goes on. The good news is that physicians win most of the medical malpractice cases in which they are defendants. However, even a victory is not pleasant for the provider when it involves a two- or three-week jury trial. This book attempts to help you avoid the process completely.

Statute of Limitations

At some point in time, is it too late for a patient to sue you? In typical lawyerlike fashion, the answer is "maybe." Limitation rules vary from state to state, but the general rule *used* to be that a patient had three years from the date of the negligence to file suit. This has been liberalized greatly by the so-called "discovery rule," which gives the patient three years from the date the patient discovered or should have discovered that you might have done something negligent. Many states have placed absolute outside limits, usually in the seven- to eight-year range, except in cases of foreign objects, where the limit is three years from detection. Some states allow children's claims up until they reach adulthood, usually age 18, and then they have an additional three years.

The latter cases, for the most part, are subject to the outside limit previously mentioned.

INSURANCE

Most state licensing boards in the United States require that you carry malpractice liability insurance in some minimum amount. There was a time when some physicians felt that if they carried no insurance, plaintiffs would not pursue them. This is highly dangerous thinking. While indeed there have been cases when an individual doctor was dropped from the case because he had no insurance, most likely, these cases did not have significant value and/or other defendants were in place. The risk of placing your personal and professional assets on the line is not worth the savings in premiums.

You should take two steps:

1. Consult with experienced malpractice insurance people in your jurisdiction to determine an adequate coverage amount.
2. Discuss with your own attorney how best to set up your practice and/or your personal assets to reduce the risk of exposure.

Once you are sued, it is too late to take those steps; doing so may be construed as an admission of liability. In other words, if a plaintiff found out that you transferred title to your home the week after receiving notice of a claim, that information may be admissible at trial as evidence of a guilty conscience.

Types of Insurance

You should also know that there are different kinds of policies. While a dissertation on insurance policies is outside of this book, following are some types of policies.

Claims-Made. In a claims-made policy, coverage is in effect if the claim is made *during* the policy period for an injury or some damages that happened *after* the policy's retroactive date. Your insurance company would not be responsible for any losses prior to the retroactive date. This can get a little complicated and should be discussed with your insurance advisor. In many states, only claims-made policies are now available.

Occurrence Policy. Coverage under an occurrence policy must be in effect when the accident or injury happens. As long as the policy was in effect on the date of the injury (for example, when medical treatment was rendered that came into question in a lawsuit), the policy would provide coverage *regardless* of when the claim is presented. If you had an occurrence insurance policy in the year 2005 and a patient brings a claim alleging that something you did in 2005 was negligent, then the policy that covered that period (i.e., 2005) would be the policy that covers that claim. If you had occurrence policy for $100,000 in 2005 and a patient files a claim against you in 2009, when you have a $1 million policy, the insurance company is only liable for up to the $100,000 limit of the 2005 policy.

If you are contemplating retirement from your practice, you need to discuss ways of providing coverage for any claims that might be brought after you leave the active practice.

Insurance Limits

With respect to the limits that you should carry, there are many schools of thought. Given the climate and the relative severity of cases and the increasing dollar amount of jury verdicts, my suggestion, subject to local advice, would be that you obtain the highest and best limits available within the jurisdiction where you practice.

Excess Policies

Your excess, or "umbrella," insurance on your home or automobile does *not* cover you for any professional liability claims in almost all circumstances. Note, however, that some nursing or allied professionals who have individual and hospital-based insurance may have additional protection from their individual policy.

RISK MANAGEMENT

In the Office Practice Setting

Good office practices can minimize the likelihood of medical legal claims. Many medical malpractice insurers provide consultation to office practices in ways of minimizing, reducing, or even, in some cases, eliminating risks of claims. For example, CRICO/RMF, the Harvard teaching hospitals' insurer, is very active in issuing patient safety strategies and continually collects recommendations from practices about how to minimize patient injuries and reduce the possibility of human error. Probably the major recommendation has been the use of electronic records or manual tracking systems. Offices can, for example, have health-screening tracking systems that monitor screening and prevent patients from slipping through the cracks. Some systems track missed appointments and generate lists of patients overdue for an appointment every two to four weeks that can be reviewed by the practice manager and providers. Obviously, in a small practice, it falls upon the individual practitioner to establish policies, preferably written, to assist in avoiding errors.

In the Hospital Setting

Almost all hospitals and clinics have risk management professionals who love to give advice on avoiding claims within the hospital setting and even in the office setting, if you only approach them. It is also very worthwhile to attend a risk management program or seminar periodically. A few hours of prevention might prevent your practice from being disrupted for weeks with a malpractice lawsuit.

Continuing Education

Most states require continuing medical education credits and some documentation of attendance—check your local requirements. You should also keep a record in your office of the continuing education programs that you have attended and even some of the materials. I have often heard plaintiff lawyers ask doctors about the continuing education courses they have taken in the past several years, and it is helpful to have that information readily available.

NATIONAL PRACTITIONER DATA BANK

What Is It?

The National Practitioner Data Bank (NPDB) is a clearing-house of information relating to medical malpractice payments and adverse actions taken against practitioners' licenses, privileges, or even professional society memberships, as well as eligibility to participate in Medicare/Medicaid. It's intended to produce information to assist in making determinations about granting clinical privileges, hiring, allowing affiliation, or licensing. Very broad in its scope, it covers physicians, dentists, and "other healthcare practitioners," including chiropractors, mental health counselors, dental assistants and hygienists, dieticians, emergency medical technicians, nurses, optometrists, pharmacists, physician's assistants, podiatrists, clinical psychologists, social workers, radiology technologists, acupuncturists, and athletic trainers.

What Is Reported?

When NPDB was going into effect, there was considerable controversy over the requirement that any and all payments made on a medical malpractice claim would be reported to the data bank. It was strongly argued that there should be some threshold so that small nuisance claims could be disposed of merely as good business decisions and not be reported. This argument did not win the day, however, so *all* payments are reported to the Data Bank. When a reportable event occurs—and before the hospital, for example, forwards a report to the Data Bank—the practitioner should review it for accuracy and content. If you feel that the report as filed is inaccurate, you have to contact the reporting entity and request that it file a correction. If it refuses to correct the report, you may then add a statement to the report or initiate a dispute. Your statement, which is limited to 4,000 characters, including spaces and punctuation, becomes a part of the report so that people accessing the Data Bank will receive the original report and your statement.

You should file a statement as an addition to a report of a payment, if the reporting entity has not already done so, in cases where there are so-called "high-low" agreements. Often in cases involving devastating injuries to a child, the parties enter into this type of an agreement. Under these provisions, even if a jury returns a verdict in favor of the doctor, saying that the doctor was not negligent or did not cause the injuries, some sum of money would be paid to the injured party. The payment, under the existing rules, would be reportable to the Data Bank. If you find yourself in such a situation, you should take steps to ensure that the terms of the agreement are in the report; this way, someone inquiring will know that you had a favorable verdict even though money was paid.

LICENSING/REGULATORY BOARDS

Most states require some type of registration of most health and affiliated professionals. From what I have seen, the number of cases of complaints before regulatory boards has increased dramatically. Bear in mind that most of these boards are consumer oriented with the objective of protecting the public. Most complaints are initiated by the patient, lawyers, the media, and sometimes by public agencies such as the police or social services. The general procedure is for the complaint to be referred to an investigator of the agency and a letter to be sent to the physician. It is strongly urged that you get help in drafting a timely response to such letters. A careful and detailed response may defuse the process in its early stages. Your malpractice insurance policy usually will pay for the assistance of an experienced healthcare attorney in drafting a response to inquiries from regulatory bodies.

We have seen a large number of regulatory complaints involving surgeons who have left operating rooms before the completion of a procedure. One reportedly left to perform another procedure, leaving the case in the hands of a very senior resident; the other left to deliver a lecture after having done the significant parts of the case. We all know that these practices occur from time to time in a busy surgical practice, but you need to be aware of the potential for a complaint. The regulatory board may believe that the patient never was told that you would not be present during the entire procedure.

Responding to a Complaint Letter

If you receive a complaint letter from a patient, you should contact your insurer for assistance in responding directly to the patient's concerns. You need to keep in mind that your response may ultimately be used against you in the event that the patient takes this a step further and makes a formal claim. Your response should be crafted carefully so it cannot be used against you in potential litigation.

Chapter 2

Office Settings

PATIENT RELATIONS

I feel obliged to report some general comments I have heard from many patients who have filed lawsuits over the years. One of the most frequent complaints is that people are kept waiting on the telephone for an inordinate amount of time before someone helps them. They also frequently complain about the general unfriendliness of the telephone contacts. Another source of concern is what appears to be a lack of concern for confidentiality when the staff person on the telephone talks about the medical condition of the patient after identifying the patient out loud, presumably within the hearing of others in the office, including waiting patients. One perspective appeared in the May 8, 2008, *New England Journal of Medicine;* entitled "Etiquette-Based Medicine," the two-page article is by Dr. Michael Kahn, who is a psychiatrist at Beth Israel Deaconess Medical Center and an assistant professor of psychiatry at Harvard Medical School. Dr. Kahn reports patient complaints about doctors "never smiling," "not listening," and, therefore, not being "respectful" and "attentive."

Build a Relationship of Trust

I have seen many, many cases where a physician or other health provider was *not* included in a lawsuit because of the personal feeling of trust the patient had for that particular doctor, even though to our review, that physician probably should have been involved in the lawsuit. A patient who is satisfied with a provider will rarely bring a lawsuit and will have a high level of understanding and tolerance in the event of human error. Therefore, I strongly recommend that you read the above commentary by Dr. Kahn, where he urges providers to have "good manners." One particular suggestion he has in the hospital setting is that you "sit down" when talking with the patient. I know of a very busy neurosurgeon in the greater Boston area who told me that his hospital had surveyed patients of the Neurosurgery Department and he continually ranked highest in patient satisfaction. One of the comments of the patients was that he spent more time with them. When I spoke with the doc-tor, he told me that his very simple way of achieving this good impression with the patient was to sit down at the bedside or next to the chair of the patient, touching them in an empathetic fashion when appropriate and looking them in the eye. He told me that he probably spent less total time with patients, but because of his approach, the patients were left with the impression that he had truly made contact with them and had spent more time with them than some of his colleagues.

Keep the Waiting Time Down

Efforts should be made to try to improve the scheduling of patients so that they are not kept waiting, sometimes for hours, in the physician's office. At the very least, if a pro-vider is running way behind schedule, a patient should be told that as soon as she shows up for her appointment and given the opportunity to reschedule. I fully recognize that with third-party payer problems and difficulties in seeing a certain number of patients in the course of a day that stay-ing on schedule can be very difficult. The use of electronic scheduling, particularly electronic medical records, can help you to take advantage of the limited time you have with the patient. In most settings, patients are seen first by an assistant to the provider, then by the provider herself. It doesn't help your image or increase the satisfaction of the patient if you appear to be hurried and harried. This again is reason why you should take a few moments to sit down with the patient, listen to him, and probe a bit with respect to his complaints. Patients could be notified prior to a scheduled appointment that they are to bring with them the following written lists:

- All current medications
- Problems they seem to be having
- Any questions they might have

By bringing in lists, they won't forget to convey this vital information in the short time that you have to spend with them. Notifications could be generated electronically as a form that would go to the patient along with the appointment notice.

Ensure Good Communication with Patients

Let me relate a brief personal experience regarding communication—or lack thereof. I consider myself to be a relatively informed patient, particularly after spending so many years involved in medical legal litigation. In any event, I was scheduled to have a relatively routine thyroid scan. Before showing up for the administration of a radioactive isotope to be followed the next day by a scan, I was never told—at least not that I remember—that I should avoid shellfish or any other food items that might contain high levels of iodine. Because of the times that these events were scheduled, I had to leave the office in the middle of the day. A technician, who had some English limitations, asked if I had eaten any fish recently. This happened to be on a Tuesday, and I said that I had eaten flounder on Saturday evening. She then checked with someone and told me that the flounder was not a problem but that shellfish might present a problem. She left, and I then realized that we had gone to a holiday buffet where I'd eaten at least six or seven shrimp. I told one of the people at the desk, who disappeared for a few moments, went down the hall, and came back to tell me that it was all right—it was not a problem. In preparation for receiving the isotope, I made a comment to the same woman technician that I was glad I remembered that I had eaten shrimp. She expressed surprise and said that the individual who had come down the hall had told her that I had "fish," and that she already knew that. She spoke with the radiologist and both the isotope and the scan on the following day were canceled and needed to be rescheduled. If I hadn't mentioned the shrimp again, I assume that the test would have gone forward and the results may have been affected. The above story is a very minor example of how small communication errors can lead to anything from a mere inconvenience to significant problems. This particular cancellation probably could have been avoided by the following steps:

- A brief information sheet could have been mailed to patients scheduled for certain kinds of testing, advising them of items to be avoided.
- The physician ordering the test could have told me to avoid shellfish, or whatever other things I was supposed to avoid, for some period prior to having these tests.
- When the person behind the desk conveyed the information to the technician (which is where the misunderstanding occurred), the

technician should have pursued the conversation a bit further.

Patients have a certain obligation to take care of themselves and ensure that they are giving the provider accurate information. Communication is indeed a two-way street. You should never discourage a patient from asking questions or seeking information about any matter involved in their medical care and treatment, even though you may think it a nuisance. Many patients, I am told, arrive with Internet searches of their symptoms, including recommendations for treatment and even medications to be prescribed. There is a great deal of information "out there." There is no way you can prevent this practice, and overall, it is beneficial to the physician-patient relationship for your patient to be well informed. You might consider directing patients to reputable resources, such as PubMed (*www.pubmed.gov*), UpToDate (*www.uptodate.com*), or your hospital website.

Good communication means fewer malpractice claims.

TELEPHONE AND EMAIL ENCOUNTERS

Keep Excellent Records

Telephone advice is a daily practice in all of your lives. I cannot emphasize enough the importance of keeping accurate records of telephone encounters with patients that involve giving any kind of advice. We had a case a number of years ago in which a pediatrician, the pediatric group, and an office nurse were sued in a medical malpractice case. A toddler had been seen the previous day with a fever. It was reported that the mother called the office the next day and told the nurse that the child now had a rash all over his body. The nurse, according to the mother of the child, advised that she should continue with the liquid antibiotic that had been prescribed and call if he wasn't better the next day. The nurse claimed that she had told the mother to bring the child in if the temperature was above a certain level and not to wait, but there was no documentation of the telephone call.

Another unfortunate case, both for a newborn and a very excellent pediatrician, involved a youngster who was discharged from the hospital with a mildly elevated bilirubin result. (We have seen more of these cases since the admission time has been cut for newborns.) In any event, the plan, according to the pediatrician, was to have daily bilirubin tests done until the bilirubin level went down. The pediatrician's planned course of action was probably above the standard of care for the average pediatrician in this practice, since the level was only mildly elevated. The doctor remembers speaking with a family member on a Friday of a holiday weekend and reminding that person to bring the child in for additional testing on Saturday. He was told by whomever he spoke with that Saturday was inconvenient and they would bring the child in on Sunday. On Sunday of the weekend in question, the pediatrician was notified of an abnormally high bilirubin level and advised the parents to take the child immediately to a specialty hospital to have the level rechecked and, if it was verified, to get immediate treatment. The parents requested that the test be done locally. Upon hearing of the double-checked level at a local hospital, the pediatrician instructed the parents to bring the child directly to the specialty hospital, where he was admitted.

The child suffered permanent hearing loss as a result of the elevated bilirubin. During the hospitalization, the parents told the pediatrician that they had driven for some time on Saturday with the child in their automobile, which prompted the investigation into the automobile deodorizer, since it was now discovered that the child had G6PD deficiency. The pediatrician also learned that the baby had been placed on a newly cleaned and deodorized carpet in the home. We had experts who were willing to testify that the chemical agent used for the cleaning of the carpeting contained Benzine, a known oxidant. Our experts from a number of fields were prepared to and, in fact, did testify at a protracted trial that it was normal to have elevated bilirubin in the first few days of life and that the child's bilirubin levels were actually within normal limits. They also testified that it was not a departure from the standard of care to fail to screen for G6PD deficiency in the early postnatal period. They also testified that even if the bilirubin had been checked on the Saturday of the weekend in question, it was probably before this child was exposed to the oxidant that caused the high rate of bilirubin found the next day.

The real sticking point in the case was the lack of documentation of the telephone discussions with the parent or family member. The person with whom the pediatrician claimed he spoke was not identified, he could not remember who it was, and—again—the name was never documented. After the jury had deliberated for several days, the insurance company negotiated a settlement of the case because of the potentially high jury verdict for a child with a permanent disability. This was a most disheartening case for all because the pediatrician was a very competent individual who acted above the standard of care; only the lack of documentation led to the result.

Train Your Staff

People in your office should be trained in handling telephone calls, handling dissatisfied patients, and having a positive and friendly attitude toward the people who call. Calls that are put on hold should be monitored so that people aren't lost, and the voice options when your telephone is answered should be kept to only a few. The patient's privacy should be kept in mind when having a telephone conversation, and you should be able to confirm the identity of the patient. In some cases, it may be appropriate to have an office manual for staff as to how they should handle routine questions and how they should document matters. Also, staff should be able to advise patients that the provider will get back to them in the latter part of the day. Telephone logs should be kept for as long as you maintain medical records. There should be provisions for handling telephone lab reports, particularly those that are exceedingly abnormal or so-called "panic values," which need to be relayed to the provider immediately. Some telephone message pads create a duplicate so that one telephone message can be inserted in the patient's record and the book of messages can be retained for a reasonable period of time. Even though it is inconvenient, I would recommend that the telephone message book be maintained for at least three calendar years. Answering services should be monitored periodically by you or some staff member to check on their efficiency and cordiality.

Liability for Telephone Advice

Legally, there is authority for the proposition that telephone advice may be the basis for a negligence claim. In these days of increased telephone calls, one needs to be very vigilant. The infant in the case involving telephone advice by a nurse showed up at the pediatric office with full-blown bacterial meningitis but survived with moderate, permanent disabilities. After a five-week trial, a jury returned a verdict in favor of the office nurse and in favor of an emergency room physician but was unable to reach a verdict as to the pediatrician, resulting in a mistrial. We had to retry the case; the second trial did not run as long, and it resulted in a finding in favor of the pediatrician. Good documentation might have helped to prevent this case or would have provided the resolution in the initial trial.

Telephone counseling has grown in prevalence, since providers are attempting to deal with the healthcare of so many people and are recognizing that not every question from a patient requires a physician visit. Some practices have services where nurses provide telephone advice free of charge. There have been cases of patients successfully suing providers because they relied on that advice and ended up delaying either going to a physician's office or an emergency room. Even in a telephone encounter where there is no physical contact with the patient, you are still legally responsible for getting some accurate history and giving reasonable and appropriate advice that complies with the standard of care. Even if the telephone contact between the provider and the patient is the first encounter and you have never had an actual in-person visit with the patient, the telephone call may be enough to form a provider-patient relationship for which you could be legally responsible.

Never prescribe over the phone for a new patient! Insist on a personal visit and clinical evaluation or refer the patient to an ambulatory setting. If you are giving advice to an established patient, there must be some way of accessing the patient's medical record.

Giving Advice by Email

Email advice from providers to patients is also becoming much more common and carries with it the same risks as telephonic advice. Of course, email creates a permanent record of the communications. Again, I emphasize the significance of keeping complete records of telephone encounters, as well as email advice to patients. As much detail as possible should be included in the record of email and telephone advice, creating documentation similar to that of an in-person visit.

The Importance of Protocols

A recent case involving a midwife-managed labor and delivery with physician backup led to injuries to the infant, probably occurring as part of the labor and delivery process. Both the physician, who was consulted about three times, and the midwife agreed that the fetal heart tracing was "nonreassuring." The hospital protocol for midwife management for women in labor provided that in the presence of a nonreassuring fetal heart strip, the case was to be "comanaged." The obstetrician assumed that this was a midwife case, and the midwife assumed that the doctor would be making clinical decisions with respect to proceeding to cesarean section. In any event, this is a classic example of a communication breakdown within the professional hospital setting, where there was no assurance that physicians who covered midwifery services and the midwives themselves knew the protocols for management. No periodic review of protocols ever took place within the Department of Obstetrics and Gynecology, where the written protocols were proven to be very damaging in the defense of the case.

If written protocols are applicable to any part of your practice, you must be aware of the content along with any updates. Your failure to follow an office or hospital protocol may be admissible as evidence that you were negligent. Conversely, following a protocol may be supportive of the proposition that you complied with the standard of care.

Following Up on Test Results

Frequently, hospital or outside laboratories report an abnormal test result that could be critical to the well-being of the patient. An exceedingly low hematocrit, for example, needs to be followed up, as does an elevated PSA result. In a number of cases over the years, I have seen situations where results were forwarded to a large medical practice, at least according to the records of the laboratory, but never make their way to the patient's chart. I had one situation where a very low hematocrit result went undetected for over a year and a half, until the patient presented at the hospital and it was discovered on review of his laboratory tests. One of the physicians saw the patient of one of the partners.

Thinking he would do his partner a favor because the patient had not had a general physical in a long time, this physician ordered routine laboratory work. The laboratory result came back showing a markedly abnormal hematocrit. According to the laboratory and even the office staff, the results were transmitted directly to the office printer. No paper results ever appeared within the patient's office chart. The hospital laboratory records indicated that the results were emailed to both the primary care physician and the physician who ordered the test. The ordering physician remembered seeing the results but knew that the patient had an upcoming appointment (which happened to be later canceled) and also noted that he had been referred to a urologist (although it turned out that the referral was for kidney stones). Nothing further was done until both physicians received a summons and complaint. A case such as this is almost impossible to defend; all that remains is to determine how to allocate insurance payments on behalf of the two physicians.

Another case involved a PSA test result that had apparently been misfiled. The office procedure was that all laboratory results were to be initialed by the physician before filing. In this case, the patient's attorney obtained a copy of the record that contained the abnormal PSA report, which was not initialed. When we asked for a copy of the record, we received no PSA report. This case was settled from the separate insurance policy of the group practice on the basis that it was a "systems error," not negligence of the physician. Because of this, the settlement was not reported to the NPDB as a payment of behalf of the provider.

A suggestion would be that any time lab tests are specifically or routinely ordered, a tickler system (either manual or electronic) should pull the patient's chart within a reasonable time (two weeks or so) to check if the lab results have come back. A simple system like this can not only help ensure good patient care but can also be perceived as an excellent preventive measure. Some electronic systems will automatically flag abnormal reports. Again, a rather elementary tickler system to track pending lab results with the assurance that they made their way to the chart, the ordering physician, and the patient's primary care physician could have caused these lawsuits never to have been filed.

RECORDS

Notes Must Be Legible

After years of representing physicians and trying to decipher some of their hieroglyphics, I would not consider it a compliment if someone told me that my handwriting was like that of a doctor. My staff and I have spent hours upon hours trying to make sense of handwritten records, thinking that after all the years of experience we have had reviewing records we could translate pretty much anything. This is *not* always the case, as shown in Figure 1.

We have had numbers of cases where physicians could not read their *own* writing and were unable to say what the

Figure 1

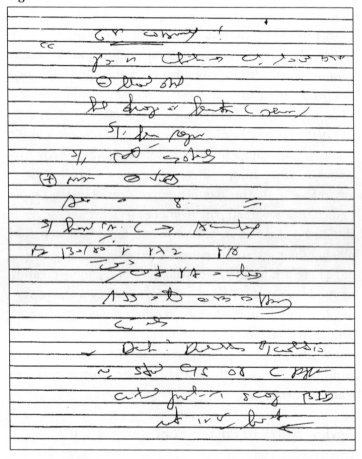

plan had been for the patient at a prior visit, perhaps a year or two earlier. This is not only embarrassing for the physician but is also not good medical care. Other situations arise where physicians or other health providers can't read the writing of a consultant or a prior or subsequent treater. It is awkward, to say the least, to be in a situation where you are defending a physician for not following a suggested course of treatment by a consultant because at the time she's questioned, she's unable to read the consultant's note. Providers cannot be expected to remember everything that happened at a prior visit or an annual visit with a patient and must rely upon the written record of these encounters.

In the hospital setting, we see more and more electronic records, which hopefully will minimize these clearly preventable errors. In the office setting, there is really little, if any, reason for having handwritten records when it is simple to dictate notes about patient encounters. Even these notes should be checked by the physician for accuracy before making their way to the patient's record.

There are hundreds of examples of legibility creating medical/legal problems—let me mention just one. We were involved in a case where an attending physician wrote an order for a patient of "15U insulin." The house officer taking off the order later interpreted this to mean 150 units, and the patient was given this excessive dose with severe consequences.

Review Notes to Ensure Continuity of Care

When seeing a patient, a good practice is to review the notes from your last visit with that patient to see if any follow-up was planned. In one case that comes to mind, a physician noted at a January visit, "Will discuss colonoscopy at 6 month follow-up visit." At the follow-up visit, however, there was no mention of colonoscopy. The physician, of course, doesn't remember the encounter, but about 18 months later, the patient was diagnosed with colon cancer and filed suit against the primary care physician. The patient testified that a colonoscopy was never mentioned.

Write Letters to Patients

For whatever reason, providers seem to resist the practice of writing letters, particularly to a patient. The few minutes that it takes to send a letter to a patient briefly describing your visit, findings, recommendations, and future plan would be well rewarded by the patient's impression of your professionalism and concern for her. The letter also serves as further documentation of your care and is made part of the patient's record. Thus, it helps to eliminate those difficult situations where the doctor says, "I must have told him *abc*, because that is my customary practice," but the patient says, "I was never told anything." Even when you refer a patient for a specialty consultation and you receive that report from the specialist, a follow-up letter, which includes lab results and so forth, should be sent to the patient. Often, a very brief note followed by just sending copies of test results with a handwritten notation on them that they are normal or good is, again, reassuring to the patient and helps to maintain a beneficial physician-patient relationship.

Electronic Records

The *New England Journal of Medicine* reported in its July 3, 2008, issue that electronic health records have great potential to improve healthcare and save time for physicians. It went on to report that physicians have been very slow to adopt these systems or to put them into effect. The article discusses a collaborative study involving a large number of practices, and I strongly recommend it for your reading pleasure and, hopefully, to encourage you to bring your practice up to the 21st century, as long as it is economically feasible.

Advantages of Electronic Record Keeping. A system that will email you abnormal test results and give you instantaneous information regarding drug interactions, all of which are highlighted in an electronic record, can be a great advance for patient safety and a wonderful time-saving device for you in a busy practice. This applies to both the office and the hospital setting, and it may be that hospitals will be slightly ahead of the curve in switching to the electronic or digital record than will offices. Although only a small minority of physicians in the United States use the electronic or digital record, those who do report a 90 percent satisfaction level with these aids.

In the fall 2008 *Harvard Public Health Review,* the cover story was "Will Digital Health Records Fix U.S. Healthcare?" To see the best and clearest example of the WHO guidelines and the 19 point safety checklist, which have been reported to not only reduce mortality rates but complication rates as well, and should lend to reducing potential malpractice cases, see *Harvard Public Health Review,* Fall '08 p. 9.

The recent U.S. presidential election saw both parties promising to make additional funding available for electronic health information systems. This is, in part, prompted by the astronomical, rapidly escalating cost of healthcare. Some experts feel that switching to computerized records may be an essential element in national healthcare reform and will result in substantial decreases in costs. In these trying economic times, you should expect rapid moves towards electronic record keeping. In fact, President Obama has made this a cornerstone of his plan to reduce overall healthcare costs.

Hardly a day goes by that some news isn't reported in the media, including the Internet, dealing with healthcare. As this book goes to press, a survey of primary care doctors is being reported. They indicate that they feel overworked, and nearly half plan to cut back on how many patients they see or leave medicine entirely. Of the 12,000 physicians surveyed, 60 percent responded that they would not recommend medicine as a career. The survey indicates that 90 percent of the responders reported that nonclinical paperwork has increased in the past three years, directly causing them to spend less time with each patient. A large number of the physician responders reported that they are working at "full capacity" or they are "overextended and overworked." According to the analysis of the survey results, electronic medical records might go a long way to saving time and reducing costs.

Electronic records are touted as leading to fewer medication errors and, as pointed out in the *Harvard Public Health Review* article, ready availability to guidelines for patients' diagnoses, even highlighting treatments that the patient is not presently receiving. A system that automatically warns you of potential side effects or interactions of a drug or its relationship to other drugs the patient currently takes clearly could reduce claims. The risk of losing documents and data when a patient receives healthcare at other locations or is transferred should be eliminated by ready access to an electronic record. Obviously, security and confidentiality need to be assured at the highest level. Pending legislation will provide grant money to encourage the adoption of these kinds of systems, giving $3 of grant money for every $1 expended by providers, and it's even keyed toward "small, non-profit, and rural healthcare providers, and for practices that will link to a network of multiple providers" (*Harvard Public Health Review* 2008, pages 6–13). Two Case Western Reserve University Professors, Sharon Hoffman at the Law School and Andy Podgurski at the School of Engineering, have co-authored "Finding a Cure: The Case for Regulation and Oversight of Electronic Health Record Systems," which is expected in the 2009 *Harvard Journal of Law and Technology*. The authors will advocate the need for street governmental regulations to assure maximum privacy of patient data, usability and interoperability. Stay tuned for the upcoming debate.

Also interesting is a recent article in the November 24, 2008, *Archives of Internal Medicine* entitled "Electronic Health Records and Malpractice Claims in Office Practice." This survey of over 1,800 Massachusetts physicians indicated that physicians who used electronic health records (reportedly about one-third of Massachusetts physicians) had a 6.1 percent history of paid malpractice claims compared with 10.8 percent of physicians without electronic records. The study covered the period of June 1, 2005, to November 30, 2005; we can assume that people have become more adept with the technology since then and these numbers will improve, leading to fewer cases and lower overall healthcare costs. A wonderful bonus for us all!

Disadvantages of Electronic Record Keeping. There are some pitfalls to electronic records. In some cases, the provider modifies stock entries. If a minor mistake is made at the outset, it generally will continue to find its way into every electronic record going forward. Periodic checking of patient histories is important to ensure the accuracy of the electronic record. A few other issues have arisen with regard to these types of records. How do you correct an error? We know what to do with a written error but not necessarily a digital one. Some systems (so I am told by my technically skilled associates) may not have that capability. In others, you may or may not be able to trace when an error was corrected, who made the change in a particular record entry, and how it may have been communicated to others. These are just things to be mindful of as you go forward, prompting questions you should ask when considering an electronic system.

After I thought I had finished this section regarding electronic records, I read the 753-page medical record of a patient who died at a major tertiary care center after having been transferred from an outside hospital. The final event for this patient involved difficulty establishing femoral access, leading to a perforation and excessive bleeding. The records indicate that the attending and surgery department were paged stat, but this being sometime after midnight, their response was delayed. What will be difficult to justify is the entry *after* the substance of the dictation indicating that the patient arrested and was pronounced dead. The postprocedure assessment was as follows: "Sedated ... resting comfortably, no complaints. Called RN for transport." ("Resting comfortably" indeed!)

Obviously this is a stock electronic form for placement of a pulmonary artery (PA) line, and the postprocedure assessment was never corrected. It's embarrassing when you encounter entries like this in a record in a serious case, but such entries are one of the pitfalls of electronic record keeping.

Also, some electronic records are difficult to follow when they are reduced to print. At least some are printed with the most current on top, which is fine, but occasionally a partial note, instead of continuing on the next page, shows up on the prior page.

We have also encountered cases where the pagination of the record changes depending on the date printed. This creates problems in your office or in court where you are referring someone to a test result that happens to be on a different page on their copy.

Just the other day, in a mock trial/focus group, we witnessed "jurors" thinking that an X-ray, which was the subject of the claims, had been reviewed by another doctor and a nurse. The entry after the X-ray report was "Reviewed by Jane Doe, R.N.—reviewed by John Simple, M.D." The nurse and doctor had reviewed *only* the report, *not* the film, but this wasn't clear.

Lastly, we spoke recently with an expert reviewer who was highly critical of our client for taking almost two months to arrange a specialty referral for a child. When we explained how this record was produced from an electronic base, he realized that he was looking at a prior encounter date, and the referral had actually been made within 24 hours.

Despite some "glitches," these records will get better as they gain more universal acceptance.

Requests or Subpoenas for Records

Always bear in mind that provider/patient communications are confidential and the unauthorized release of patient information may expose you to liability. When a patient requests copies of records, you should be certain that you have a completed authorization form from the patient authorizing the release of records to her custody. Always provide copies; *never* send originals. If a patient's attorney requests records, you should be certain that you have correspondence indicating that the individual is the attorney for the patient and that you receive a completed authorization form signed by the patient, dated reasonably current (usually within 30 days), authorizing the release of her records. You are not obligated to provide any report or interpretation of the records in question, and if asked to do so by the patient or his attorney, you should be clear in your understanding of the purpose for their wanting such a report.

Fees. Do *not* charge excessive fees for records. Some states' licensing boards have regulations limiting the cost for duplicating records to $0.25 per page. In any event, be reasonable. Some attorneys send along an applicable regulation when they make a request for records so that you can refer to it when determining how much to charge. It is probably inadvisable to charge a patient directly for a copy of her records unless they are voluminous. I've heard patients in lawsuits say that they were shocked at their physician actually charging them for a copy of their own records. Even though doing so may be justified, it isn't worth the aggravation and the possibility of antagonizing a patient.

Responding to a Summons for Records. If you receive a summons for production of records, you should ask your risk manager or representative of your malpractice insurer about the correct policy regarding your response. You may have some records that are specially protected, such as HIV results or testing, psychiatric records, and other highly privileged information. The mere fact that you receive a summons for records does not necessarily mean that you have to comply blindly with it.

Once you are satisfied that responding is appropriate, your office should contact the requesting attorney and ask whether she is only looking for records so that you can avoid any personal appearance. If you are informed that the attorney requires your personal presence, you should contact your malpractice insurer and discuss the need for legal representation at such a deposition. Often, issues can be resolved by telephone calls between an attorney appointed to represent your interests and the attorney seeking the information. More often than you can imagine, providers, unrepresented, have gone to depositions to answer questions about their patients and ended up being added to the case as a codefendant. While it is no guarantee you will not become a party to the lawsuit, representation by counsel will ensure appropriate preparation for the process and protect your rights.

Because of HIPAA requirements, you should review the summons for records to see that there is an affidavit from the party seeking the records; that the party has given the patient, through the patient's attorney, an opportunity to object to the production of the records; and that no objection has been made. If you have any concerns, you should contact the patient directly to tell him of this request for his records.

Responding to a Request for Opinion or Testimony. If you receive a request for information or medical opinion with respect to a patient, be cautious with regard to commenting on the prior care for the following reasons:

- You may not know all of the facts surrounding the treatment rendered.
- If you document criticism of a patient's prior care and treatment, you will probably be subpoenaed to give deposition and/or trial testimony if the matter is put into suit.

If you receive a request to provide expert testimony, be aware that you do not have to serve as an expert witness in any matter, unless you want to. Should you choose to serve as an expert witness, you are entitled to be compensated for your time. As an expert witness, you may have to appear as a witness at a trial, if the case is not resolved earlier.

On the other hand, you cannot ignore deposition subpoenas. You could be sanctioned by the court for ignoring a deposition subpoena, including fines and even more severe penalties in some extreme cases. Again, if you receive a deposition subpoena that calls for your presence for purposes of testifying, contact your insurer and request legal counsel for this deposition. Your appointed counsel will prepare you for and accompany you to your deposition. He may be able to arrange for the deposition to be taken at your office and/or at a time that will be minimally inconvenient to you.

Avoid Blaming

When you are making entries in records, be extraordinarily cautious about "blaming the other guy" or "casting stones." Never criticize others without knowing all of the facts, and even in those circumstances, be prudent. Any notation by you as a subsequent treater, based on a cursory review of a patient's records and without necessarily knowing all the circumstances of the earlier treatment efforts or the reasons behind an earlier treatment plan, not only can be embarrassing to you at a later trial, when it is shown that you were unaware of the underlying facts, but can be most damaging to one of your colleagues, who may end up being unfairly involved in prolonged medical malpractice litigation. Remember that you would not want your own conduct to be second-guessed by someone who is not in possession of the full facts of the patient's situation.

For example, I saw a case where a woman, who had undergone genital surgery, presented to the emergency room of a large hospital saying that she had been to her surgeon, who had performed a procedure in an office setting. She said that she had seen him just an hour earlier, and he had told her to go home. When the young female was seen by attending gynecologists, they were outraged that a physician would have sent her home, because she needed to be hospitalized to care for a very large hematoma and possible infection. They reported this to the Patient Safety Committee, and the hospital ended up reporting the physician to a licensing board. What apparently happened was that the surgeon who performed the in-office procedure had actually told the patient to go to the emergency room of the hospital, which was very near his office, although he had no hospital privileges. Not knowing all of the facts created a nightmare for a surgeon.

Altering Records

Never alter any record of any patient! The few times that we've had cases over the years where a physician or someone under her direction has changed a record, doing so has resulted in an absolute disaster for the client. It is one of the few unforgivable mistakes a provider can make. In the very popular movie *The Verdict* (which was based on an actual case, part of which I actually saw as a very young law student), the allegation on behalf of the plaintiff was that the obstetrician, anesthesiologist, or someone at their direction had changed the time of the patient's last meal (the patient had aspirated), making it substantially earlier than the original entry in the record. A very prominent handwriting expert testified in the case that the time had been altered by a physician who had made other entries in the particular record, leading to a large verdict against the physicians.

In a more current case, a physical therapist whom we were representing was being prepared for her deposition testimony. She had made notes of the visits by a patient who had been referred by a hand surgeon, such as he had "alcohol on his breath," was "drunk," and other disparaging remarks. These statements may very well have been true. Regrettably, the plaintiff's lawyer had a clean copy of the record, obtained before the lawsuit began, which had none of these entries. The physical therapist told me that the doctor had called her with the request that she make those notations in the record. I reported this to the attorney for the doctor and to the insurance company, and the case ended up being settled.

If you find yourself in a position where you have to make a change to a record, you should just draw a line through the entry or entries so that they still can be read and make the notation "error." You may then proceed with an additional or corrected entry, but it should be dated to show that you have done this before having any inkling that someone might bring a claim. This same procedure would apply to any addendum to a record. It should be carefully documented as to when the addendum was made and the purpose for doing so, and addendums should never be done after you have received a notice of a claim.

THE NONCOMPLIANT PATIENT: DOCUMENTATION IS KEY

This must be one of the most frustrating situations for any healthcare provider: you are trying to do your best job for the patient, but the patient just doesn't listen to you. These situations, historically, have proven to be "malpractice cases in waiting."

You should exercise an even higher level of caution and documentation with respect to this type of patient. You should document her reluctance or outright refusal to follow suggestions, such as screening. A record that says, for example, "discussed colonoscopy" is absolutely no defense in a case where the noncompliant patient, who has told you that she doesn't want to have screening, ends up suing you because she ends up with colon cancer.

Again, even though it's a nuisance, you need to write the patient a letter. Sending a letter emphasizing the importance of the patient's following up your recommendations really is very helpful, probably to the patient and certainly to you to prevent potential liability. If you find that everything else has failed, you need to ask the patient to sign off on the fact that you have advised a certain course of action. I recognize that this is yet another layer of administrative duties, but believe me, it will save you problems in the future. If you have been encouraging a patient, for example, to have a screening, such as a mammogram, colonoscopy, or PSA test, and the patient is resistant, you should dictate a very brief note to the patient for the next visit, asking the patient to acknowledge that you told him about the risks and benefits and asking that he acknowledge that you have done so. The following is a suggestion of the kind of note you might ask the patient to sign:

> *I know that Dr. Blank has told me that I need to have certain testing done, such as laboratory tests, screening tests, X-rays, and other types of potentially diagnostic studies. I have told Dr. Blank that I do not want to have these done, at least at this time. He/She has advised me that getting such testing done is very advisable, yet I know that I do not want to do it at this time and assure Dr. Blank that I will get back to him/her at our next visit if I change my mind.*
>
> *Signed,*
>
> *Jody Patient*

I was involved in a case almost 20 years ago where an orthopedic surgeon treated a trauma victim with multiple injuries. An incidental finding on one of the radiology studies showed a lesion of the patient's tibia, which was thought to be benign. The patient was seen in the office in January, and arrangements were made for a follow-up in February. The patient did not show up and about two years later broke his leg skiing. Studies at that time showed that the lesion was an adamantinoma. The physician said that he had told the patient about the lesion; the patient said he was not told about the lesion. The court found that the patient was not negligent in failing to follow up and that the doctor should have taken steps to follow up when the patient was a no-show. The court felt that the doctor should have pursued the unresolved issue of the lesion when it was left up in the air due to the patient's not returning. Here we have yet another case of lack of documentation.

In a U.S. Court of Appeals case in Rhode Island, a patient in the fall of one year reported to an internist that he had been seen at a Veterans Administration hospital the prior spring and a test had shown blood in his stool. The doctor urged the patient to get the medical records for him. The doctor did not seek to obtain the medical records himself. The doctor testified that he felt that the patient was intelligent and that he had relied upon the patient to follow through and obtain the information. The patient did not obtain the records, did not communicate with the internist, and returned almost three and a half years later with stage IV colon cancer. The Appeals Court held that the expert for the patient should have been allowed to testify that it was negligent for the internist not to have pursued the records and to have followed up with the patient. Again, this is a case of no documentation of a significant discussion with the patient.

The lesson to be learned is that with potentially serious conditions,

- be certain to document what you told the patient;
- be certain to document that the patient understood what you said;
- have a system for checking on no-shows; and
- have a system for selectively sending follow-up letters to patients.

THE NO-SHOW PATIENT

This is a conundrum for any practicing physician. In a busy practice, it is really very difficult to keep track of people who don't show up. It's easy to defend a situation where a new patient does not show up but more difficult when you have an established relationship with a patient whom you know has potential problems.

Following Up on Test Results

We talked earlier about the no-show and noncompliant patient, but a few more comments are probably justifiable, considering how no-shows can lead to potential lawsuits. Above, we discussed a situation where the patient's file showed an abnormal PSA result and the follow-up appointment apparently had been cancelled by the office staff, not the patient. This lapse clearly presents problems for the office practice; staff should have had some type of procedural safeguard to ensure that the patient was aware of an abnormal result.

Incorporate this axiom into your professional life: *If you order a test—you own it.* Many reviewers who have looked at cases such as this one for us have felt that a physician who orders a test, even if not having an established relationship with a patient, should follow up if the test result is abnormal. Even someone who didn't order the test, who is covering for the primary care physician and receives one of these abnormal results, should be obligated to follow up with the patient. A telephone call with very careful documentation may be adequate, but again, I fall back on the old axiom that "if it's written, it's defensible." A simple, short note to the patient that he has an abnormal result that needs to be followed up, which includes a brief explanation and does not terrify the patient, is good medical practice and a very good way to prevent potential claims. Other situations with respect to no-show patients have been mentioned earlier, but if you have any kind of outstanding issues with any patient and he fails to appear for a follow-up appointment, you at least need to address the issue by letter.

Other Matters Requiring Follow-Up

Many trauma surgeons deal with people who have essential need for follow-up, and although they explain that to patients, those discussions don't get documented thoroughly enough. There may be one follow-up visit in the office and arrangements for additional follow-up, and then the patient is "lost." To protect you and to provide good medical care for the patient—again, I come back to the old adage of "putting things in writing"—a simple letter can prevent a myriad of problems. Just writing a letter to the patient, with a copy to the file and/or any other care provider involved, can ensure that the patient will indeed follow up and protect you years down the road if the patient decides that the failure to follow up was your fault and on your watch.

TERMINATING THE PHYSICIAN-PATIENT RELATIONSHIP

After receiving so many telephone calls from care providers over the years on this issue, and given our litigious climate, I think that physicians, in spite of their obligations to patients, need to address seriously when it is appropriate to terminate the physician-patient relationship. Patients terminate this relationship all the time by just never showing up again. You need to look at situations where a patient is obviously being so difficult, so noncompliant, and so resistant to treatment recommendations that it is almost impossible for you to deal with them. Such situations may involve personality conflicts, difficulties with staff, or a vast array of problems.

The relationship between you and a patient depends on faith and a degree of confidence. When circumstances, and there may be many, affect your ongoing ability to provide quality care, it is appropriate that the relationship be terminated. Following are some examples of situations that justify termination:

- Patient obtains drugs illegally.
- Patient threatens injury or other harm to you, staff, or other patients.
- Patient engages in inappropriate behavior in the office setting.
- A general breakdown in communication occurs, resulting in extreme difficulty in providing quality care.

You have a legal right to terminate this relationship, which is based on contract. However, you need to be cautious.

Procedure for Terminating the Relationship
I would suggest the following procedure:

- Check any local regulatory provisions that may control termination.

- Check with your local medical society regarding potential ethical concerns.
- Be aware of potential limitations in third-party payer agreements.
- Have a particular concern with impact of the Americans with Disabilities Act on how you handle any disabled or handicapped patient.

You should also do the following:

- Provide some explanation for ending the relationship.
- Give the patient ample time to find another provider (30 days, for example).
- Offer to treat the patient for a reasonable period to allow the patient to obtain another physician.
- If possible, offer some assistance to the patient in finding another healthcare provider.
- Document the termination appropriately in the medical record.
- Obtain authority from the patient to send a copy of the medical record to the new physician.

I would suggest sending the patient a letter along the following lines:

Dear Jody Patient:
Because of your continued failure to follow my treatment recommendations [other reasons may be inserted

here], which in my opinion affects your general health and well-being, I feel that it is difficult for me and members of my staff to provide you with good quality care.

I do not believe that it is in your or my best interest that I continue as your physician. I will not be in a position to act as your healthcare provider after [30 days from the date of this letter].

I encourage you to arrange for another healthcare provider as soon as possible. We, of course, will provide your new provider with a copy of your medical records.

In the event of any emergency, you should go to the nearest emergency room. We are also prepared to assist you in any emergency situation.

If you have problems in finding another provider, you should contact [local or state medical society].

Sincerely,

Blaine Blank, MD

In some extreme situations, you may feel a patient truly poses a risk to you or others in your office. You should seek private counsel in this regard, but a more strongly worded letter telling the patient that he should no longer visit the office premises and, as of a certain date, that you will consider a visit to be trespassing may be appropriate. Sending such a letter makes the situation somewhat easier should you need to call local law enforcement authorities.

Remember: The reason you give for terminating the relationship should be tempered carefully with your awareness that patients have the right to make their own decisions about treatment and lifestyle.

AVOID GIVING GUARANTEES

Don't promise to cure a patient or give an overly optimistic assurance of the outcome of any particular treatment. If you go too far, your assurance may be part of the basis of legal action if the results aren't achieved. Some plaintiff attorney firms routinely include claims for breach of warranty and guarantee, because they might win a case against you even if they don't have an expert to support a departure from the standard of care. The temptation to engage in such comments is great, particularly in the cosmetic area, where the patient has expectations of a particular result and is often shown "before" and "after" digitally produced pictures. It is okay to be cautiously optimistic, but don't go overboard. Be wary of ever telling a patient that she is having a treatment or a procedure that is "simple," because it may turn out not to be simple. Be careful telling a patient that you are doing a "routine" procedure, as not all such procedures turn out to be routine. Don't tell a patient that "no complications" will occur, because they do indeed occur, often when least expected.

CONSENT

Informed consent over the years has been part of almost every malpractice case we have defended. If the plaintiff can make a jury of laypeople believe that the physician didn't disclose adequate information to the patient about a particular procedure, it's a large step on the way to proving liability, and it doesn't usually require the testimony of an

expert to show that a reasonable physician would be aware
that what happened was a recognizable risk of the procedure. Extremely remote risks are generally not required to
be disclosed, but as the level of potential severity rises, so
does the obligation to disclose to the patient.

How to Ensure Adequate Consent from Patients

Patients have the right to be told what to expect and to determine what will be done to care for their health, and their
decisions may not always be in agreement with your judgment. Ideally, discussions about consent should build trust
and confidence and reduce the shock and disappointment
of an adverse event. If you treat a patient without his consent,
then legally you have committed an assault and battery for
which you absolutely would be liable. If a patient refuses to
sign a consent form, you should go no further but rather
should explore further whether the patient fully understands the process. This can be done by additional meetings
with the patient or with the aid of interpreter services, when
appropriate. It is also useful to have another family member
of the patient's choosing present for any discussions. If you
believe that the patient's refusal to consent is due to a lack
of competency, you should document that refusal and your
opinion with respect to competency, and you should contact
your risk manager or the legal department of the hospital
where the proposed procedure was to be performed.

Whenever possible, the consent should be explained
by the physician who is to do the procedure. I know that in
large teaching institutions, procuring consent is frequently
delegated to house staff. It certainly makes us nervous about

defending these cases when there is no documentation that the attending physician had a discussion of the consent process. There should at least be a notation in the record that the attending who is to perform the procedure, even if she is doing so with the assistance of a resident, went over the consent form and reaffirmed the discussion between the patient and the house officer.

With respect to consent, you need to be aware that in most states, the test of whether consent was given is a subjective, patient-oriented test and not what the doctor thinks is best. It is truly the patient's right to choose; your obligation is to comply with that right by having a duty to disclose information that an average patient would consider important in the decision-making process, not necessarily what you as a physician might think is important.

Written Consent Forms

I am from the school of thought that strongly supports having written consent forms. There was a time when there were different theories and some institutions departed from the written form and encouraged physicians merely to make notes in the patient's record. We look at consent differently, because we see these cases years later when a patient is claiming that he was never told about any of the risks that regrettably have occurred. Studies have documented that patients who have had the risks of procedures thoroughly explained forget that they were even told those risks (even with documented witnesses) after a short period of time. My recommendation, therefore, is that whenever possible, there should be a written consent form.

This consent form should describe the key potential risks of the procedure. In a recent case we tried, the patient had a sigmoid colectomy resulting in an "injury to a ureter," leading to the loss of a kidney. I was hopeful that the consent form (knowing that the institution required a written consent) would contain "injury to the ureter" as a potential risk or complication. Unfortunately, the form only said that the patient was consenting to a "sigmoid colectomy." No risks or complications were listed. The office record of the surgeon did contain a note that he discussed the possibility of damage to "adjacent organs," but since injury to the ureter would be relatively high on that potential list, it would have been much more helpful had it been specifically mentioned. As it turned out, the case was really tried on other grounds (which we will talk about later) because of medical record problems leading to complications in the defense of this case and hospital records that probably initiated the whole case.

It would be impossible to include all risks on the consent form. The ones included should be based on the severity of potential harm and the likelihood of its occurrence. Even a small chance of death or serious disability is significant enough to mention in the consent form. Likewise, the more common complications should be mentioned, even if they are relatively minor. It really isn't a very good defense to a case for a physician to say, "Well, I told her that the procedure might cause death, but I didn't tell the patient that the procedure might damage a ureter." This is particularly true when the patient can show, through evidence, that the risk of death might have been 1 in 1,000,000 and the risk of injury to the ureter 1 in 10,000.

If house staff or assistants are to be involved in the procedure subject to the consent, their participation should be outlined on the form as well and explained to the patient.

When Patients Decline to Give Consent

Numerous legal decisions around the country have dealt with the issue of informed consent, particularly when it relates to people who decline to give consent on religious grounds for what would appear to be an absolutely necessary lifesaving procedure. The greatest difficulty arises when you are dealing with parents of a minor or a handicapped person who are making these decisions on behalf of the patient. You need to obtain legal advice from either a hospital attorney or your own attorney before either acceding to the wishes of the guardians or going forward with treatment. Classic examples concern Jehovah's Witnesses in cases where they decline blood transfusions or use of blood products. I have seen situations where anesthesiologists in certain hospitals have said that they felt that it would be unethical for them to let a patient die because they would not accept blood products and have told surgical staff that, regardless of the wishes of the patient, they would administer blood products if they felt doing so was necessary to save a patient's life. Some tertiary care centers now have procedures for the surgical treatment of Jehovah's Witnesses without the use of blood products and will agree to accept these patients in transfer. Be aware of how you can transfer these patients to appropriate institutions.

A number of years ago, I received a call on a Saturday from a surgeon whom I had known for a number of years, telling me that he had a patient with severe necrotizing pancreatitis who needed surgical debridement of the pancreas. The husband of the patient wanted her to have the surgery to save her life. The question was whether we needed to go to court for permission since the patient was a Jehovah's Witness and blood products would obviously be needed. Ordinarily, one would need to have a court hearing for substituted judgment for the patient. I got the call on a weekend, and the situation was already emergent. I knew from past experience that it would take at least the balance of that day and maybe into Sunday or Monday to assemble the appropriate team, including judges, guardians, a court-appointed lawyer for the patient, and so forth. The doctor told me that he thought that this was truly a lifesaving procedure. More importantly, he told me that he had asked the patient if she wanted to live and, before she was intubated, she had told the surgical team that indeed she did want to live. According to the surgeon and the staff, a notation was made of this on a plain piece of paper and initialed by the patient.

She was taken to surgery, had several debridements, had blood transfusions, survived, and then, of course, sued the surgeons for saving her life and for violating her constitutional rights by the administration of blood products. Naturally, the first thing we went looking for was the statement from the patient regarding her desire to live. Because this documentation was out of the ordinary and didn't look like a usual hospital record, it was nowhere to be found. Partly because we were unable to produce that documentation, the case went forward and proceeded to trial after a few years of a drawn-out discovery process and a very unpleasant lawsuit.

A jury returned a verdict very quickly in favor of the surgeon and the surgical resident.

These cases are particularly sensitive, and we will discuss them in different areas as we go forward. Providers have to realize that sometimes notations, written on pieces of paper that are given to a physician or nurse or other support staff, could be critical to the future prevention or defense of a malpractice case. How they end up being lost is only a matter of conjecture. There must be more diligence in maintaining records, including nontraditional records.

Remember: Be vigilant in obtaining appropriate consent from patients. Also, be sure to communicate with any close family members who appear to be involved in the care of the patient, even though they are secondary and the choice is truly the patient's, not theirs or yours. Keep the signed forms.

CURRICULUM VITAE

Periodically (I would recommend annually), check your curriculum vitae (CV) for accuracy.

What Not to Include

Resist the temptation to include nonmedical matters, such as being a member of a country club or holding some world book of records award for running on a treadmill. (I have actually seen these entries in CVs.) Likewise, try not to "puff up" the CV too much. I have had interesting cross-examinations of experts who, in trying to overreach a bit, included entries such as the fact that they had taught "dog

surgery" and had written articles regarding lactic dehydro-
genase (LDH) adaptation in goldfish. Likewise, social memberships, such as a "member of the Burlington Country
Club," the fact that you had a "hole in one," or that you were
an "outstanding student at a summer math camp" may contribute a bit of humor in the courtroom but not to your
credibility. The humor will be at your expense. I am not
being facetious. I recognize that some of this information
may have legitimate scientific value, but it is cannon fod-
der for examination in a courtroom. Try to look at some
of these entries with the anticipation that a layperson may
look at them and think about what the reaction might be
to them.

The ultimate sin with respect to CVs is to indicate that
you are board-certified when you are not. I have seen this
happen to an expert or two over the years with devastating
results. Sometimes you need to be aware of what may be on
a hospital website with respect to your involvement at the
institution. For example, if you have indicated that you do
5,000 of a certain procedure and the website of the institution indicates that the institution as a whole, with four other
physicians in your speciality, only does 5,000, that can be
embarrassing in court.

Your Internet Profile

In this day and age, you also need to be very careful with
what information you put out on the Internet. Plaintiff lawyers are inventive and are very good at digging into your
public professional profile. If it's out there on the Web, they
will know. Very little that you do or say on the Internet is

private. If people try hard enough, they will discover that you may very well be the host of a particular blog with discrediting opinions posted on it. In other words, be careful in *all* of your communications with respect to your medical practice.

A recent medical malpractice case appeared to be going relatively well, until the physician was on the witness stand. The lawyer for the plaintiff discovered that the doctor was the creator of a blog dealing primarily with his distaste for malpractice lawsuits and actually talking about the case that was on trial. She took the defendant doctor by surprise by asking him on the stand if he was Doctor X, the creator of the website, sometimes referred to as the Ghost Writer. He had made highly derogatory remarks about the plaintiff's lawyer and the validity of her case. The revelation was so damaging to the overall defense of the case that it settled out of court the next day. You can imagine the drama in the courtroom when these comments made by the doctor on trial were disclosed.

Again, you have to use your head. Be cautious and conservative and never do anything about a patient or a potential case without seeking outside advice. You may not necessarily be the best objective judge of what happened in the course of a patient's treatment. Often, it is best to say nothing, particularly on the Internet.

REFERRALS

When you refer a patient to another physician, it should be clear who is responsible to schedule the appointment with the consultant and whether there is any urgency to doing so. As the attending physician, you need to provide the consultant with sufficient records and information and a clear question or questions as to what areas you would like the consultant to address. The consultant needs to have an adequate system for communicating findings back to the attending, particularly to communicate abnormal findings timely. Both the attending and the consultant should take care not to make disparaging comments about other clinicians in the course of their correspondence. As the attending, you need to know, after a referral, precisely what the consultant has done and whether a careful discussion of risks and alternatives for a given course of action has taken place.

We had a situation where a young man of moderate mental disability came with his father to a visit with the primary care physician with complaints of testicular pain. He was seen by a nurse practitioner, but the actual testicular exam was done by the attending. It was felt that he needed to be seen by a urologist. It was the end of the day, and the office attempted to call to arrange an appointment with the urologist but was not able to do so. The office claimed that it gave a referral card to the patient's father with instructions that he was to call the urologist to make an appointment. There was never any follow-up to see if this had been done. Lack of documentation—yet again—became a factor in the case, as the patient and his family claimed that they were not told to contact the urologist. Regrettably, about one year later, the patient was diagnosed with testicular cancer. Fortunately, he had a reasonably good result subsequent to surgery.

This case points out the importance of being very careful to document who has the responsibility of obtaining the referral and following up. Again, you have the responsibility, as a primary care physician, to see that a planned referral actually takes place and, if not, why not. Believe it or not, claims have been made where a patient has alleged that her primary care physician referred her to a consultant who was not qualified to treat her condition, and a court has found liability for referring the patient to an unqualified specialist. You should periodically rethink the list of people you use as referrals to assure yourself that they are still the people to whom you would wish to send your patients for particular problems.

CONFIDENTIALITY

We talked earlier about how to respond to requests for information and to subpoenas for records and/or your presence at depositions. The general rule is that you should never talk or write about a patient to anyone who may be in an adversarial position to the patient without your patient's permission or all parties being present, as would be the case in a deposition where your patient is represented by counsel and a physician or other party who is being sued is likewise represented by counsel. Whenever in doubt, you should obtain advice from risk management and/or legal counsel. You should not respond to telephone requests for patient information without the patient's written permission. Be aware of institutional and state-mandated policies regarding release of information related to psychiatric care,

substance abuse, HIV, or other areas specially protected
by law.

Times and Places to Exercise Particular Caution

Public Venues. Everyone sees the postings in hospitals, particularly in elevators, advising people not to talk about
patients in public. This should be stressed within your office,
including at your office's reception desk. It is really not a
good practice for you to walk a patient back to a waiting
room and announce in the presence of other people who
are waiting to be seen your plan for future action relative
to the patient. This should be done in confidence and, of
course, be documented.

Answering Machines. Often when you return a telephone
call from a patient, you will encounter an answering machine. It is not recommended that you leave any kind of
clinical information on the machine, because the machine
may be accessible to people other than the patient. You
should leave your name, the time you called, and a return
number at which you may be reached and/or your office
number, with the indication that you are returning the call
of the patient and nothing more unless the patient has
asked you to do so.

Minor Patients. With respect to minors (i.e., patients under
the age of 18), except in unusual circumstances, such as
when the minor is pregnant, you need to have parental con-

sent before you release any information. Likewise, in what can be a very difficult situation for a physician, you need to have the authority of a person over the age of 18 for releasing information, even to the patient's parents. You should be very diplomatic in involving the young patient, particularly one who is still living in the parental home or still being supported by parents, in his medical decisions. We all understand why parents would not want to be divorced from the medical care of their child. At the same time, we must respect all patients' privacy and confidentiality. With a bit of time, a careful and mutually satisfactory middle road can be worked out so that the young person and the parents are content with how you handle the care and the sharing of information.

Young Adults. We have seen cases where college students of age 19 or so have committed suicide after lengthy psychiatric consultations with student health services. In almost all of the cases resulting in lawsuits, the parents were never made aware of these extremely dangerous situations involving their children. If you wish to avoid the anguish of a case like this, you must persuade your young patients to give permission to share information with their family members, who are paying their tuition and still supporting them. Perhaps students should be told on admission to college that they are expected to sign an authorization to release medical information to their parents in high-risk situations. The right of privacy shouldn't trump the potential of death or serious injury to a child or young adult.

When Reporting Is Required or Ethical

Harm to Self or Others. Despite an obligation to confidentiality, you are required to report certain conditions, such as communicable diseases, or when you feel that the patient is a danger to herself or to others. The classic example is a California case known as *Tarasoff v. The Board of Regents,* where a psychiatrist was sued for failure to warn people whom the patient had clearly identified as potential targets of violence. Such cases are now an exception to the general rule of confidentiality.

The *Tarasoff* case deserves a deeper look, because it triggered other legal decisions across the country, as well as action by many legislative bodies to amend or modify the usual rule of confidentiality. Confidentiality is a particularly sensitive issue in the therapist-patient relationship. Even a family physician, and certainly a specialist, should evaluate a patient who is undergoing a crisis as to their potential risk for homicide or suicide. In this foggy, difficult area without a great deal of diagnostic criteria, a physician really has no other path than to speak with the patient and ask about his thoughts and intentions to harm himself or others.

It is beyond the scope of this book to discuss what factors should be taken into account in assessing a patient for suicidal or homicidal risk, but if you clinically feel that a patient is suicidal, then the patient needs to be hospitalized. In some circumstances, that needs to be done by involuntary commitment to a psychiatric ward or a psychiatric hospital. If you clinically feel that the patient has real homicidal intention directed at identifiable victims, you need either to hospitalize that patient or, according to the majority of states, you have a duty to warn and take steps to protect the intended victims of your patient. To avoid potential liability, as we have seen in cases involving mass murders at schools and colleges, you need to err on the side of public safety. This can be difficult for some physicians who feel very strongly about confidentiality, but in looking at the issue from the viewpoint of potential liability, it would be much easier to defend you for a breach of confidentiality of a patient when you had, in your judgment, a reasonable basis for notifying law enforcement officials, school officials, a spouse, friend, or other identifiable person of a potential risk than, on the other hand, to defend you in a case where someone, or large numbers of people, have been killed or maimed.

The *Tarasoff* case itself involved a young University of California—Berkeley graduate student who met a young woman named Tarasoff at the International House at the university. The couple apparently kissed on New Year's Eve, and the patient, Mr. Poddar, who was from another culture, interpreted the kiss to mean the existence of a serious relationship, which was not the intention of the young woman. She told him that she was not interested in entering into any kind of intimate relationship. As a result, the patient became depressed, neglected his studies, and finally began being treated by a psychologist at the school. He told the psychologist that he intended to kill this young woman. The psychologist requested campus police to hold Mr. Poddar and that he be committed. He was detained but shortly afterwards was released by the psychologist's supervisor. No warning was given to this young woman or her brother, who was also a student, or any other member of her family. Several months later, Mr. Poddar killed Tatania Tarasoff. The court found that the doctor had a duty not only to a patient but also to individuals who are specifically being threatened by a patient. The court stated, in referring to the confidentiality of the physician-patient relationship, "The protective privilege ends where the public peril begins." This ruling has been pretty much followed throughout the country, and you need to be fully aware of it.

Licensing Board Investigations. What do you do if the licensing board in your state is investigating another physician for some conduct where you were one of the subsequent treaters? In some situations, you may have precipitated the complaint to the licensing board by bringing it to the attention of the hospital risk manager, from where it went to a patient safety committee and the hospital filed the actual report. In some situations, your patient is not the person complaining to the licensing agency and, in some circumstances, may not wish you to disclose any confidential information you may have obtained as the treating physician. Reporting an incident of subpar healthcare by another provider and assisting the licensing agencies in their investigations generally will give you some immunity in any claim for breach of confidentiality and to a claim by the other health provider, as long as you have acted in good faith. If you are asked to meet with representatives of a licensing board who are going to be presenting evidence in an adversarial trial involving the physician who may be subject to discipline, the wise course would be to request a signed release of information from your patient. Local and state laws may permit you to have these kinds of prehearing discussions, but be alert for potential problems. Your primary ethical and legal responsibility is to maintain the confidentiality of the patient and your role in the patient's care.

Obviously, if you are contacted by an attorney representing the physician who is the subject of a complaint or that physician himself, you should strictly insist upon a signed release and/or the presence of a legal representative of the patient. This is true even if you as a provider may feel that the physician who is the subject of a potential hearing did not do anything wrong. This is a classic situation where you need to contact a risk manager at your institution or your malpractice insurer to obtain advice and potential representation before trying to weave your way through this field of potential legal landmines.

Patient Rights

There is an old legal axiom that for every legal "right," there is a corresponding "duty." In other words, if a patient has a "right to privacy," then you as a healthcare provider have a "duty to protect that privacy and confidentiality." Likewise, if a patient has a "right to a copy of his medical record," then you have a duty or obligation to provide that copy. Many of you are familiar with the fact that if you act as a "good Samaritan" in rendering uncompensated care to someone in an emergency situation, you can only be held liable for gross negligence. A person in an emergency situation has no right to expect that you will treat him, and you have no corresponding duty to treat that individual. Therefore, the law provides a certain degree of protection when you act in the best traditions of medicine by assisting a person under those circumstances, and you will have very limited liability.

If you are careful, you can avoid ever getting into a conflict with a patient over any of these issues.

HIPAA Requirements. To further complicate your existence, Congress enacted the Health Insurance Portability and Accountability Act (HIPAA) of 1996. HIPAA essentially mandates minimum privacy standards for patient records. States may have more rigid privacy requirements but not less. Like most federal legislation, it has given birth to large numbers of regulations, which are extremely difficult to follow and to implement, particularly in a small practice. Essentially, when in doubt, seek a written authorization from your patient before releasing information.

We have encountered many problems in cases where we are defending a physician and send a subpoena for records. We have to include an affidavit that we have complied with HIPAA by notifying the attorney for the patient. In almost all cases, the patient's attorney does not object to our acquiring the records for use in a lawsuit. Sometimes, we even have a letter from the patient's attorney assenting to the release of the information. In spite of this, we have been told by some hospitals and some providers that they will not disclose or release their records without the written permission of the patient. The more we try to simplify matters, the more complicated they become. HIPAA has certainly been overinterpreted to insert a number of obstacles to what should be a reasonable flow of information, particularly for use in defending a healthcare provider. You need to be aware of the law and the corresponding regulations. Most information is available at the U.S. Department of Health and Human Services website (*www.hhs.gov*).

COLLECTING UNPAID BALANCES
CAN TRIGGER LAWSUITS: IS IT WORTH IT?

I, personally, am a great believer that we, as professionals, are entitled to be paid for our services. Given all of the complexities of billing, including dealing with multiple third-party payers, getting paid can become challenging. You should be very careful in your collection techniques, however. There is absolutely nothing wrong with pursuing a patient for the balance on a bill that remains unpaid and/or uncovered by a third-party payer, provided that plan is not one under which you have agreed to accept its payment as payment in full. That aside, you should place limits on how far you will go. I have seen a number of cases where collection agencies, which are the next step up from intra-office billing, have irritated and aggravated patients so much that they have brought a lawsuit when they would not have done so had a bill not been pursued so aggressively.

Sometimes, if two or three requests for payment go unheeded, it may take nothing more than a simple telephone call to the patient to ask what the problem is and if you can do something to resolve any disagreement. Frequently, you can avoid future problems by simply writing off a relatively small balance. I am not attempting to interfere with your business practices but merely making a suggestion of how to avoid getting into some unnecessary litigation. I have certainly seen cases where collection agencies have filed suit against a patient, which is met by a countersuit for medical negligence, opening a "can of worms" with which you really don't want, or need, to deal.

A tragic case in Ohio some years ago involved a young patient who had been admitted to a psychiatric unit with a diagnosis of major depression. Shortly after admission, her treating physician ordered her discharge from the hospital. At about the time of discharge, the hospital's financial officer contacted the patient, in the hospital, regarding payment of her hospital bill. She left the hospital and committed suicide that same day.

The administrator of her estate sued the financial officer of the hospital, saying it was negligent conduct to approach the patient regarding payment of the hospital bill, taking into account her fragile situation. Part of the reason the case did not go very far was that the plaintiff had only an affidavit of a licensed clinical psychologist, which was conclusory and didn't raise a genuine issue for trial. There was nothing to show what the accepted practice for a hospital should have been in approaching a psychiatric patient concerning payment of the bill.

I look at the case as one of true insensitivity and an open invitation to a lawsuit. Sometimes you need to conduct your business and your practice as a compassionate human being.

If this family had engaged more competent representation, this could have been a very compelling case before a jury of laypeople. Don't ever do something this dumb!

Chapter 3

Hospital Settings

TYPES OF HOSPITALS

Before discussing staff privileges, committees, and peer review, a little background information would be useful. In the United States, there are, generally speaking, three types of hospitals:

1. Charitable institutions, which account for about 50 percent of facilities

2. Governmental hospitals, whether they be local, state, county, or federal, which account for about 38 percent
3. For-profit hospitals, which account for about 12 percent

The nature of the hospital where you may have privileges can have some impact on your potential liability. (Note that in this section, I am speaking in generalities, because a discussion of all 50 states' laws is outside the scope of this book.)

Charitable Hospitals

Most charitable hospitals have some type of limited liability, usually with a dollar cap on a recovery against the facility. In states with this type of provision, lawyers for patients will generally sue the physicians, ancillary staff, and employees, because they are not subject to the charitable limitation and most, if not all of them, are insured.

For-Profit Hospitals

With a for-profit hospital, on the other hand, there is generally no limit on the dollar amount that can be recovered. It is also easier, in relative terms, for a patient to receive a money award when suing a corporate entity. In many of these circumstances, plaintiff lawyers will sue only the institution, because doing so takes the personality of the physician, nurse, or technician out of the equation, leaving only the corporation.

Governmental Hospitals

With governmental hospitals, a plaintiff generally cannot file a suit against a true employee of the governmental hospital. Governmental hospitals vary from state to state, but with respect to federal hospitals, such as those of the U.S. Department of Veterans Affairs, these hospitals are covered by the Federal Tort Claims Act (FTCA). Someone who qualifies as an employee of the federal hospital has personal immunity. The federal government, however, is liable without any limitation on the dollar amount of recovery. To somewhat compensate for this, FTCA cases are tried with no jury.

STAFF PRIVILEGES

Staff privileges in a hospital, as a general rule, are available to physicians, dentists, podiatrists, nurse midwives, and other allied professionals, depending on the bylaws of the facility. Because of the increase in paperwork involved in medical staff applications, most institutions have gone to appointments that are valid for two years. Whatever your staff status may be, you should be sure to check the privileges for which you apply every two years, as well as the ones that are granted, so that you are confident over the next two years that you are not operating or performing procedures outside of the scope of your privileges.

Categories of Staff

Active Staff. These professionals regularly admit patients or regularly provide services for patients in the hospital or in the community served by the hospital. Most institutions provisionally appoint active staff for periods such as six months until the appointment is approved. Active staff members generally have a number of responsibilities, such as attendance at meetings and service on committees.

Courtesy Staff. Generally, these individuals meet the qualifications for full staff privileges but admit only a small number of patients during a calendar year. Often, these individuals are on the full staff of another accredited hospital and serve the provisional period at the hospital where they applied for courtesy staff privileges.

Consulting Staff. Generally, these physicians are already members of the medical staff or, more likely, are from another hospital and possess certain clinical expertise and come to the hospital when scheduled or when asked to render a consultative opinion.

Associate Staff. Generally these are individuals without a hospital practice but who provide services for patients in the community served by the hospital. This category is becoming more common in the day of hospitalists, where a primary care physician or other doctor may admit a patient but not necessarily be the physician following up on the care in the hospital. This practice, of course, needs to be explained to the patient.

Honorary Staff. These practitioners have served as members of the staff and, because of their reputation and contribution to the facility, are continued in the category of honorary. The privileges and prerogatives of the honorary member are subject to the bylaws of the institution. Often, they are allowed to serve on medical staff committees and vote but generally are not required to pay dues.

Management Roles and Potential Liability

The reason that I have described the various categories and provisions for hospital staff is to increase your awareness of what kind of hospital you may be affiliated with and some of the peculiarities of potential liability. Cases have arisen around the country of physicians who have voted to not grant staff privileges to a competing group practice. To avoid embroiling yourself in some unnecessary litigation that, while it may not be medical malpractice, can be equally drawn out, you should exercise discretion and not participate in votes that present a potential conflict with your personal and business interests.

If you are a committee member or up a little bit in the membership echelon, you should inquire as to whether the institution will add you to its liability policy for these types of management functions. Some medical malpractice insurance policies provide this kind of coverage, but there is such wide variance that you need to check within your particular jurisdiction. This would apply to the for-profit hospital situation as well. Generally speaking, governmental hospitals provide immunity when you serve in some kind of staff capacity.

A number of states have laws that provide immunity for medical staff committees in the profit or nonprofit setting, provided that you are serving without compensation. The only potential for liability would be if you acted in a grossly negligent fashion (for example, by knowingly credential-ing a recognized incompetent physician) or for intentional acts.

A notorious case in the late 1980s was *Ross v. Beaumont Hospital.* The case revolved around a surgeon who had narco-lepsy, which caused her to fall asleep at inopportune times, including during surgery. The surgeon was 300 pounds and 5 feet 2 inches tall. This resulted in problems with her knees, which caused her to use a walker and sometimes even a wheelchair. The main source, however, of concern was that she was extremely abusive to nurses, other physicians, patients, and their families. The hospital finally terminated her medical staff appointment and clinical privileges. She sued the chief of staff and the chief of the department of surgery, as well as the hospital, on the basis that they had dis-criminated against her because of her sex, her narcolepsy handicap, and her weight. You would think that these kinds of things don't happen, but they do. A jury initially found that there had been discrimination and awarded substantial damages. In a civil rights case like this, however, the finding of the jury is only advisory. The federal judge then found that the termination of the doctor's appointment did not take place solely because of the handicap of narcolepsy and dismissed the case.

There was little the administration could have done to avoid this claim. The real key to the defense of this case was the excellent documentation of the more than 50 inci-dents of disruptive behavior and abuse. When serving on committees or in some other administrative capacity, you really need to be aware of whether decisions are being made in the best interest of the hospital or being based on self-interest. Acting in your own self-interest to the detriment of another physician who does not have all of the extraordinary circumstances as Dr. Ross might expose you to antitrust liability.

PEER REVIEW

Peer review is the process of doctors evaluating the quality of the practice of their colleagues to ensure compliance with generally accepted standards. Depending on the institution, peer review committees are involved in the initial credentialing and ongoing review of a doctor's performance and scope of privileges during the renewal process. State licensing boards are also involved in overseeing physician's standards but not to the extent of hospital peer review.

Peer Review and Liability

A number of articles in the medical and legal literature have been published with respect to peer review, defending it as an effective means of self-regulating the profession. Most state legislatures and the federal government have enacted laws that protect peer review committee members from liability, and the work product of the committee is generally exempt from discovery in a legal action. The strong public policy favoring open peer review outweighs the general rule of things being available for discovery. As long as you are participating in the peer review process and you act without malice and in good faith, you have immunity from civil liability.

The peer review process, when it works the way it is intended, is designed to help minimize occasions of medical malpractice by openly and candidly discussing the quality of a physician's care within the hospital setting. This, in and of itself, should help to minimize claims by preventing minor incidents from growing into major ones.

Review of physician privileges should be made without participation by competitors of the reviewed physician, if possible. It may be necessary to retain outside peer review from a retired physician, a medical school faculty member, or a qualified quality assurance consultant to avoid the appearance of conflict of interest, especially in a medical setting.

MISTAKES

Another recent development has been notification from Medicare and other third-party payers that they will no longer pay for certain "mistakes." Can you imagine the patient who has a procedure done at a hospital and some weeks or months later receives a notification from the third-party payer that it has not paid the hospital because of a surgical site infection or pulmonary embolism? These are among some of the so-called "errors" for which Medicare says it will not pay.

The National Quality Forum, a nonprofit healthcare safety agency, has issued a list of 28 avoidable errors, and states are adding to these rapidly. The list of errors is as follows:

- Surgery on the wrong body part
- Surgery on the wrong patient
- Wrong surgical procedure performed on a patient
- Foreign object left in a patient after surgery
- Death of a generally healthy patient during or immediately after surgery for a localized problem
- Patient death or serious disability associated with using contaminated drugs, devices, or biologics
- Patient death or serious disability associated with the malfunction of a device
- Patient death or serious disability associated with intravascular air embolism
- An infant being discharged to the wrong person
- Patient death or serious disability associated with the patient disappearing for more than four hours (whatever that means)
- A patient's suicide or attempted suicide resulting in serious disability
- Patient death or serious disability associated with a medication error
- Patient death or serious disability associated with transfusion of blood or blood product of the wrong type
- Maternal death or serious disability associated with labor or delivery in a low-risk pregnancy
- Patient death or serious disability associated with the onset of hypoglycemia

- Death or serious disability associated with failure to identify and treat hyperbilirubinemia in newborns
- Severe pressure ulcers acquired in the hospital
- Patient death or serious disability due to spinal manipulative therapy
- Patient death or serious disability associated with an electric shock
- Any incident in which a line, designated for oxygen or other gas to be delivered to a patient, contains the wrong gas or is contaminated by toxic substances
- Patient death or serious disability associated with a burn while a patient in the hospital
- Patient death associated with a fall suffered in the hospital
- Patient death or serious disability associated with the use of restraints or bedrails
- Any instance of care ordered by or provided by someone impersonating a healthcare provider
- The abduction of a patient
- Sexual assault on a patient
- Death or significant injury to a patient or staff member resulting from a physical assault in the hospital
- Artificial insemination with the wrong donor sperm or donor

The list of 28 items from the National Quality Forum has not been accepted in most states. Medicare has its own list of "errors" for which it won't pay. At least five states have adopted this controversial list of 28, however, and other states have chosen not to reimburse for a number of errors. Utah, at the moment, lists some 31 potential errors for which it will not make payment.

This rush not to compensate hospitals for procedures that are problematic can cause nightmares for healthcare providers. Just imagine the patient receiving the notice from the third-party payer saying, "We have declined to pay for your procedure, which cost $10,000, because it was based on a medical error." I would think that this would send the patient rushing to the nearest medical malpractice lawyer. As of this writing, at least five states have agreed to waive fees for these 28 "errors" identified by the National Quality Forum. I am going to talk about some of them individually, because they really do not meet the standard definition of deviation from the standard of care. Obviously, if your patient receives notification from an insurer or a governmental agency that is has declined to pay for part of a hospitalization because of an "event" or "error," your patient may well sue you.

Just because something happened that is on one of these lists does not necessarily mean that the healthcare provider committed negligence or departed from the standard of care. The whole concept brings back memories of what I mentioned earlier about the doctrine of *res ipsa loquitor*, meaning that just because an event happens, it equates with negligence. Some of these incidents are really precipitated by the physician. For example, a physician might knowingly perform wrong-sited surgery, such as doing a right-sided hernia when the documentation called for left-sided hernia, and bill the patient for doing both sides. This borders on stupidity, and if you do this, you really need to wake up and be aware of what is going on in your practice and with your billing practices.

Types of Mistakes

Wrong-Site Surgery. Hospitals have taken great strides to try to prevent this type of event by implementing strict procedures including the initialing of operative sites by the surgeon and calling for "time-outs." We did have a recent case where this procedure appeared to be followed but still resulted in problems. Surgery took place on a very young child at a well-known pediatric hospital. The surgeon had initialed the operative site high on the point of the proposed incision. When the surgical team got to the operating room and followed the procedure of a time-out, the patient had already been draped, and it was difficult to see the markings for the operative site. In any event, things proceeded to the second time-out, and then the surgeon began the procedure. Only when the anesthesiologist was relieved by a certified registered nurse anesthetist, did the replacement notice that the operative permit was valid only for the opposite side. She brought it to the attention of the scrub technician, who brought it to the attention of the surgeon, and the procedure was stopped. The surgeon went out and discussed the situation with the family and asked if they wanted him to stop or to proceed to correct the side which needed surgery. They went ahead with the surgical procedure and have had a reasonably good physician-patient relationship since then.

Investigation revealed that, in spite of this elaborate time-out procedure, people did not stop to assess where they were at in the course of the procedure and what was going on. Although a time-out was called, the staff just continued with their normal routine. Time-outs call for rigid enforcement, particularly by the operating surgeon, to insist upon compliance with the protocol, which will protect all participants from the potential of a lawsuit for wrong-site surgery.

In the *Harvard Public Health Review* of fall 2008, there is an article about how millions of errors worldwide could be avoided by using checklists. Dr. Atul Gawande, a wonderful patient safety advocate, a surgeon at Brigham & Women's Hospital in Boston, and someone I always enjoy reading, whether it be in a medical journal or in the *New Yorker* magazine, advocates the use of checklists. The article reproduces the World Health Organization safety checklist shown in Figure 2 on the next page. See the January 29, 2009 *New England Journal of Medicine* special article "A Surgical Safety Checklist to Reduce Morbidity and Mortality in a Global Population," which reports that use of a 19-item surgical safety checklist (based on WHO guidelines) resulted in the rate of death dropping from 1.5% to 0.8% and the complication rate dropping from 11.0% to 7.0%. Strong evidence included that simple checklists work!

My example above shows that these measures can be in effect but staff don't necessarily follow them. Using a checklist is as simple as it could possibly be, as long as people

Figure 2

SURGICAL SAFETY CHECKLIST (First Edition)

World Health Organization

Before induction of anaesthesia ▶▶▶▶▶▶▶▶ Before skin incision ▶▶▶▶▶▶▶▶ Before patient leaves operating room

SIGN IN

☐ PATIENT HAS CONFIRMED
- IDENTITY
- SITE
- PROCEDURE
- CONSENT

☐ SITE MARKED/NOT APPLICABLE

☐ ANAESTHESIA SAFETY CHECK COMPLETED

☐ PULSE OXIMETER ON PATIENT AND FUNCTIONING

DOES PATIENT HAVE A:

KNOWN ALLERGY?
☐ NO
☐ YES

DIFFICULT AIRWAY/ASPIRATION RISK?
☐ NO
☐ YES, AND EQUIPMENT/ASSISTANCE AVAILABLE

RISK OF >500ML BLOOD LOSS
(7ML/KG IN CHILDREN)?
☐ NO
☐ YES, AND ADEQUATE INTRAVENOUS ACCESS
AND FLUIDS PLANNED

TIME OUT

☐ CONFIRM ALL TEAM MEMBERS HAVE
INTRODUCED THEMSELVES BY NAME AND
ROLE

☐ SURGEON, ANAESTHESIA PROFESSIONAL
AND NURSE VERBALLY CONFIRM
- PATIENT
- SITE
- PROCEDURE

ANTICIPATED CRITICAL EVENTS

☐ SURGEON REVIEWS: WHAT ARE THE
CRITICAL OR UNEXPECTED STEPS,
OPERATIVE DURATION, ANTICIPATED
BLOOD LOSS?

☐ ANAESTHESIA TEAM REVIEWS: ARE THERE
ANY PATIENT-SPECIFIC CONCERNS?

☐ NURSING TEAM REVIEWS: HAS STERILITY
(INCLUDING INDICATOR RESULTS) BEEN
CONFIRMED? ARE THERE EQUIPMENT
ISSUES OR ANY CONCERNS?

HAS ANTIBIOTIC PROPHYLAXIS BEEN GIVEN
WITHIN THE LAST 60 MINUTES?
☐ YES
☐ NOT APPLICABLE

IS ESSENTIAL IMAGING DISPLAYED?
☐ YES
☐ NOT APPLICABLE

SIGN OUT

NURSE VERBALLY CONFIRMS WITH THE
TEAM:

☐ THE NAME OF THE PROCEDURE RECORDED

☐ THAT INSTRUMENT, SPONGE AND NEEDLE
COUNTS ARE CORRECT (OR NOT
APPLICABLE)

☐ HOW THE SPECIMEN IS LABELLED
(INCLUDING PATIENT NAME)

☐ WHETHER THERE ARE ANY EQUIPMENT
PROBLEMS TO BE ADDRESSED

☐ SURGEON, ANAESTHESIA PROFESSIONAL
AND NURSE REVIEW THE KEY CONCERNS
FOR RECOVERY AND MANAGEMENT
OF THIS PATIENT

THIS CHECKLIST IS NOT INTENDED TO BE COMPREHENSIVE. ADDITIONS AND MODIFICATIONS TO FIT LOCAL PRACTICE ARE ENCOURAGED.

actually take time to comply with the steps. A checklist can save you immeasurable time away from patient care, in a courtroom, in the event of an error.

Suicide. I have considerable concerns about a number of the "errors" published by the National Quality Forum. For example, we have defended many cases over many years concerning suicides of patients. The question really comes down to whether the institution and/or the physician recognized the high risk of suicide and whether sufficient precautions were taken to ensure that some safety mechanism was in place. As everyone knows, it is not always possible to prevent a suicide by a patient. To include in these "errors" that a suicide should allow a third-party payer to disapprove payment is outrageous.

Deaths Due to Medication Deaths or serious disability due to medica-tion. We have seen cases where Demerol and Vistaril were given intravenously instead of intramuscularly resulting in the loss of the patient's finger and instances where patients were given excessive blood thinners resulting in serious hemorrhage. Computerized records are generally felt to reduce these "accidents." Some institutions use "bar codes" to match the patient to the appropriate medicine regimen. This area also should call for expert evaluation.

Hyperbilirubinemia. Or take the many newborns who have evidence of hyperbilirubinemia. The standard of care calls for reasonable monitoring of these levels. This has been a particular problem because of the early discharge of mothers and babies postnatally. To include this as an entry where insurers will not pay for hospital care will only generate many, many more cases and is totally unfair to the clinician.

Falls. One of the most incredible proposals that I see in these regulations is that a "fall" in the hospital may be, in and of itself, reason for nonpayment of the bill; listing falls as "errors" will precipitate many, many medical negligence claims.

Sexual Assault. Lastly, to imply that you, as the healthcare provider, should not be paid in a situation where a patient may have been a victim of sexual assault defies imagination. Unless you have been an active participant in some mismanagement of a patient that led to an assault, it is outrageous that a third-party payer would not pay you and/or the institution for your services. Obviously, the patient has recourse in bringing a criminal complaint, malpractice claim, or straight negligence claim against the people involved. Why you would be subjected to these penalties is beyond my imagination.

What Can Be Done

These situations all require careful review by independent experts after the fact. What is happening is third-party payers are trying to get off the hook from paying bills, and all these lists of "errors" will do is generate significantly more medical malpractice claims. You need to be on guard with respect to these types of claims and potential claims and make all of your legislative representatives—at the local, regional, and national levels—aware that crazy things are happening that they need to deal with.

A few minutes at your computer will be an education if you check the hundreds or thousands of entries regarding medical and hospital errors. For every one story favorable to healthcare providers, a hundred strike terror in the hearts of the average consumer. Recently, an article appeared at Forbes.com dealing with "scariest hospital risks," which included the following:

- Wrong-site surgery, which is certainly being addressed by surgeons and operating room teams with policies for marking surgical sites and time-outs
- Postoperative infections due to what the article refers to as failure to give preoperative antibiotics
- Bleeding secondary to the patient being on anticoagulant medications
- Patients getting "sicker" in the hospital (Patients with an acute situation requiring hospitalization may have an underlying condition, such as diabetes, pushed into the background and leave the hospital sicker than when they arrived. Providers need to monitor underlying and/or chronic conditions to ensure that they are being attended to as well.)
- Pneumonias secondary to the use of ventilators that collect bacteria (Hospitals have, for the

most part, developed programs to deal with potential infections from ventilators.)
- Infections secondary to use of a contaminated catheter
- Wrong medication (Medication errors should be greatly minimized by the use of computers at the bedside and in hospital pharmacies.)

Core causes of the problem, according to some experts who were quoted, are overcrowding and doctors and nurses not spending enough time with each patient. Eugene Litvak, a researcher at Boston University Medical Center, has advocated what appears to be a relatively straightforward solution: better scheduling in and of itself can reduce overcrowding and reduce surgical errors and infections. According to the article, which appeared at Forbes.com along with "Scariest Hospital Risks," admissions and operations have in the past been scheduled without regard to how many operating rooms could work at the same time. When scheduling of admissions was evened out, the number of surgeries that needed to be rescheduled in a year was reduced from 700 to 7. A more controlled flow of patients in and out of the hospital contributes to the better overall functioning of surgical teams. Instead of having downtime some days and overcrowding other days with large numbers of patients contributing to high stress levels, managing patient flow evens out the number of cases each day, reducing the stress and overcrowding that has been shown to contribute to a number of preventable errors.

PRACTICE GUIDELINES/PATHWAYS

Can any of these nightmares be avoided by the use of "practice guidelines" or "practice parameters"?

The Purpose of Guidelines

When administrators originally sought to introduce practice guidelines, they were met with great resistance by practitioners. Guidelines were intended to be recommendations for treatment methods for certain diagnoses and procedures. Doctors trained more than twenty years ago have generally been opposed to what they perceive as mandatory guidelines for appropriate clinical practice, saying that this is "cookbook medicine." Recently, physicians have become more willing to participate in the development of guidelines that have been shown to improve patient care and to eliminate or reduce medical injuries and malpractice lawsuits. As a general rule, these guidelines are written by physicians to aid other physicians in the management of patients in particular clinical settings. They have gained acceptance as "evidence based" medicine, which if most physicians follow them, truly represent what similar Doctors would do in a like situation and are strong evidence of the standard of care. Most third party payers now base their payment decisions on guidelines promulgated by the various specialty societies. The many anesthesia guidelines, which as discussed below really have become a standard of care and have greatly reduced the number of malpractice cases against anesthesiologists.

Benefits of Guidelines

These practice parameters or guidelines are generally expert judgments reviewed by competent people in your field and, if followed, may offer better evidence to a jury than the standard of care voiced by a "hired expert." They also constitute tools to assist the decision-making process. Many older physicians have expressed concerns about being restricted to "cookbook medicine," but my advice is that if you feel a need to deviate from any practice parameter, you should document valid reasons for doing so. For example, physicians prescribe contrary to the *Physicians' Desk Reference* (PDR) everyday, and doing so is not a departure from the standard of care but is left to the individual judgment of the physician. Furthermore, it would serve you well to be supportive of these kinds of programs, which will help to reduce claims against you and others in various specialties or in the primary care setting. As long as there is good communication among the physician, allied healthcare practitioners, and administration, these practice parameters are truly the tools of the future.

In some states, with Maine in the forefront, legal provisions provide that compliance with the guidelines is an affirmative defense for doctors in a medical malpractice case. In other words, if the doctor can prove that she complied with the practice parameter guidelines, this evidence would be a defense to a medical malpractice case, despite what any expert might say on behalf of the plaintiff or even on behalf of the defendant. This is a significant benefit to a defendant in a malpractice case. This is now being debated in a number of states, and I urge you to be supportive of these changes.

The practice parameters, in general, should be thought of as a considerable assistance in decision making, since they are the distillation of vast amounts of material and can be supportive of what you do in caring for a particular patient. Practice parameters are the equivalent of a review of your judgment, based upon the opinions of experts involved in the practice of medicine in your specialty, as opposed to "standards" set by the so-called "hired guns" to whom I referred earlier. Guidelines tend to be reasonable, explicit group judgments, which are not only better for patient care but are most beneficial in defending your actions with respect to patient care. These practice parameters may, in fact, decrease the amount of time that you need to spend with a patient. As long as you feel comfortable with the practice parameters, they can be extraordinarily helpful to you as a physician, as well as to the patient.

Guidelines and Standard of Care

We discussed earlier how the standard of care is established for purposes of medical malpractice. An expert for the plaintiff/patient tells a fact finder his opinion regarding the standard of care. That opinion is then countered by your testimony and that of experts retained by your attorney. In other words, the standard of care is really set by the parameters of medicine; the legal definition incorporates the generally accepted standard of care of physicians. One of the difficulties with the concept is that it is subject to the vagaries of the fact-finding system, the personalities and credibility of experts on either side, as well as your own credibility and reasonableness under difficult circumstances in a courtroom. Although we often interject medical literature into the legal process as an objective standard, it can still be difficult to overcome the natural sympathies of a jury of lay-people for a severely injured patient. Although still a work in progress, these practice guidelines, which have gradually gained acceptance, may be the single most objective way for the defendants in medical cases to show to a jury or a judge what the objective standard of care is, unaffected and unprejudiced by the fact that a claim has been brought.

I remember doing a number of presentations at different hospitals for groups who were considering having practice parameters for their particular specialty, including early efforts to have protocols or guidelines in stroke cases. The big-gest concern of clinicians was whether if they departed from the proposed guidelines, would they be considered negligent. As I understand the guidelines, under most circumstances, they are recommendations for treatment methods regarding certain conditions and procedures. They are tools to assist the decision-making process, and if you are in a circumstance where you feel compelled to deviate from the guideline or pathway, you should document carefully your valid reasons for doing so. Again, good documentation will carry the day.

Even in the presence of clinical guidelines, you still must exercise your clinical judgment. Whatever guidelines are in place should be kept up-to-date, since they deal with the dis-tillation of large amount of information. As a general rule, they should improve the litigation process for you because your judgment has been reviewed by numerous experts, outside of a courtroom, as opposed to what is sometimes referred to as "standards by hired guns."

The Example of Anesthesiology

Anesthesiologists, who used to be subject to large numbers of medical malpractice claims have, as a group, greatly reduced those claims through the use of practice guidelines, which became anesthesia standards. These protocols are the best example of the validity of the use of practice guidelines. They may hold the key to the reduction of medical costs, particularly those associated with "defensive medicine." They have had the impact of not only improving patient safety and customary practice in anesthesiology, but anesthesiologists apparently seem to have little, if any, difficulty in complying with the official recommendations of the American Society of Anesthesiologists (ASA). Most anesthesiologists consider the guidelines to be "authoritative" (something we will talk about later), and they have provided a considerable amount of protection to anesthesiologists, statistically resulting in the reduction of claims for this specialty. These guidelines constitute a useful lesson for other areas of medicine. Obviously, it would be wise to inform patients that they are going to be treated within certain recognized guidelines that have been promulgated by the literature and learned experts, and with which you agree, so that they understand the role of the guidelines in their care and treatment, including with allied professionals.

Guidelines: State by State

Some states are looking at how best to deal legally with the use of the guidelines. In an early Maine project, the procedure enacted was that the plaintiff could not introduce the guidelines in a medical malpractice case, since they were voluntary and not admissible to show a departure from the standard of care if a doctor chose not to follow them. The doctor, however, could show compliance with the guidelines as an affirmative defense. If you complied with the guidelines, you would have what we talked about earlier as the burden of proof to show that you did, in fact, comply with the guidelines, and that would be a defense to the medical malpractice claim supporting the fact that you complied with the standard of care.

The states of Florida, Minnesota, and Vermont have joined with Maine in recognizing practice guidelines as being equivalent to the standard of care on the public policy grounds that doing so will decrease the ordering of defensive medical tests by physicians and, consequently, reduce healthcare costs.

Drawbacks to Guidelines

Despite the benefits of practice guidelines, you should always recognize your fiduciary duty to your patient and not follow guidelines that you feel have only been issued to reduce costs. Rely still on your individual judgment. The sooner there is uniformity of guidelines, the better, in my opinion, for the defense of potential claims and perhaps even the prevention of filing of claims.

One of the problems in making effective use of practice guidelines is that they come from so many sources. While you may be complying with a guideline approved by the American College of Surgery (ACS), other guidelines, such as from the American Cancer Society, may contradict the ones in your specialty. Likewise, recommendations for screening for colon and rectal cancer become the subject of many cases involving guidelines, and a physician may have followed the recommendations of the U.S. Preventive Task Force (USPTS) but not the recommendations of the American Cancer Society or the Gastroenterology Society or the guidelines of some other organization. My point is that guidelines are becoming part of malpractice cases for use by both plaintiffs and defendants, and the real need is to have some legal protection for your conduct when you, in fact, follow guidelines by having uniform guidelines. You should check with your individual state as to the status of the law and any proposed legislation. Until guidelines are issued from one source, the safest route is to follow guidelines issued by your specialty.

Contrary to some of the literature, it can be quite difficult to discredit some of the "hired guns" who travel around the country testifying against physicians. These experts generally appear in the most sympathetic cases. At least one maternal fetal expert gives opinions in neurology, perinatal medicine, obstetrics and gynecology, and a number of things outside the scope of her expertise, but she has done it for so long and is so smooth that she can carry the day for severely injured plaintiffs. I have talked about this issue with jurors who were willing to speak and with focus groups, and they really don't have a problem with the fact that someone testifies a great deal, as the plaintiff's lawyer presents these people as having devoted their lives to advocating for the severely injured. (I question the validity of that assessment.)

Most jurors and focus groups also wonder why anyone gets into the issue of fees earned by an expert. If a plaintiff expert has made millions of dollars testifying, jurors I have talked with feel that this person must be indeed a "renowned expert." On the other hand, in the normal case, it would appear that experts for both sides are being compensated quite well, and it really neutralizes that issue. I have tried numbers of cases where I have agreed with the plaintiff lawyer not even to raise, as an issue, the compensation of experts for the plaintiff *or* the defendant, as the concept tends to be irrelevant.

For Further Information

The National Guideline Clearinghouse of the Department of Health and Human Services website (*www.guideline.gov*) is a public resource of clinical practice guidelines.

HOUSE STAFF

In discussing *house staff,* I use the term in the broadest possible context. At any given moment in a hospital, particularly a teaching hospital, there may be medical students, nursing students, physical therapy students, respiratory technician students, X-ray technology students, laboratory technician students, and others whom I am probably overlooking. The more professional areas of house staff would be interns, residents, and fellows. Each of these categories comes with its own set of potential liability and potential malpractice issues. This is not only for the individual, as someone still in a training situation, but also for those of you who may be supervising such individuals. People with practices who have medical students participating in patient care should check to ensure that they have adequate insurance coverage.

Students and Those Who Supervise Them

With respect to those of you who may fall within the classically accepted definition of *student*, you should double-check to find out what kind of insurance you are provided with when you are working in the hospital setting or even making home visits for a hospital program. In many cases, the school where you are a student insures you for liability, and often the liability policy of the hospital also covers you.

Students in the hospital setting are encouraged to dress professionally, complete with a white coat. To many members of the public, even though you may be relatively young, you do not necessarily appear to be a student. It is imperative that you tell a patient with whom you are interacting that you are a medical student and if they have any questions or concerns, you will see that someone in a supervisory capacity attends to them.

All individuals in training programs should consider the type of institution where they are employed or studying. We mentioned earlier that public hospitals generally provide a cloak of immunity, which would extend to medical house officers, nursing students, medical students, and other allied professionals, particularly those in training. In the for-profit hospital, again, the inclination of plaintiffs would be to bring the claim directly against the hospital because it is easier to recover a judgment. You should take affirmative steps to be assured that you have adequate insurance coverage. Again, the most important step you can take is to disclose to the patient that you are a student. You don't want an occasion to arise, as we have seen, where a patient was injured by an X-ray device being operated by a student technician and the patient's biggest complaint was that he was never told that the individual was a student. Such a lack of disclosure can make it more difficult to defend a claim against the student, the supervisor, or the institution.

As I mentioned earlier, most charitable hospitals have limited liability. In those circumstances, plaintiffs generally will sue the employees. Often, nurses or technicians are surprised when they find themselves the subject of a lawsuit, thinking that people would only make a claim against the hospital. In most circumstances, the insurance policy of the charitable hospital covers you for any claims.

Since students generally are permitted to make entries in the medical record, I urge you to be extremely accurate when documenting patient care and, again, to identify clearly your level of training in every note you write. The consequences of careless or inaccurate notes by staff in training have been the subject of hundreds of medical malpractice cases.

An Example: Documentation by House Staff

The process of preparing this book was interrupted by a very necessary diversion. I had to prepare for a case in defending a general surgeon in a medical malpractice claim also involving the board-certified assistant surgeon. The entire case revolved around many of the points that I have tried to make here. Let me give you some of the background.

The patient was an older woman who presented to a general surgeon, my client, upon referral by her primary care physician, for multiple bouts of diverticulitis. When she met with the general surgeon for the first time, he recommended and later performed a colonoscopy, since he was also a qualified surgical endoscopist. While performing the endoscopy, he noticed severe narrowing at the sigmoid colon. My client recommended to the patient that she have an elective colectomy. He explained that if it were done on an elective basis, in most cases, it would not be necessary to do a colostomy. The patient went for a second opinion at a major teaching institution, and it was decided not to go forward with surgery at that time.

One year later, she returned to my client, again with rectal bleeding and another obvious episode of diverticulitis. At that meeting, the surgeon again recommended that she have surgical correction of the problem by removing a portion of the sigmoid colon. The patient again elected not to do this. Seven months later, she presented at the emergency room of a community hospital with a question of bowel obstruction. She was given medication to try to relieve the obstruction and was sent home. Two days later, she was admitted to my client at a neighboring community hospital, which was affiliated with one of the major teaching hospitals.

My client met with the patient and her daughter to discuss what options were available at that time. Again, he recommended colectomy, but now he felt that he would probably not be able to avoid a colostomy. He did make efforts over the first two to three days of the admission to clear the obstructed colon, but those efforts were unsuccessful.

On the third day of admission, the patient had a surgical colectomy with a colostomy and had a relatively rocky postoperative course. On postoperative day nine, it was discovered that she had a urinoma, and it was recognized that there had been some type of injury to the ureter during the surgery. My client referred the patient to a urology colleague, who performed appropriate studies and planned to attempt a repair of the ureter. Several days later, the family elected to transfer the patient to a major tertiary care treatment center for further action. The discharge diagnosis, which was never disputed by my client, was an "injury to the ureter" that probably occurred during the course of the surgical procedure and was a recognized risk of this kind of procedure, particularly in the presence of dense adhesions. These dense adhesions were anticipated because of her medical history, including bouts of diverticulitis, and were also observed and noted during the surgical procedure.

Although consent never was raised as an issue at the time of trial, because, when her surgery occurred, it was in the nature of urgent or emergent, the consent form merely stated "surgical colectomy"; there was no mention of surgical risks at all in the form. (See the discussion of consent forms in chapter 2.) My client's office note did indicate that he explained in very general terms the risks of the surgery, including "injury to adjacent organs." Now, if the primary concern going into the procedure was injury to the ureter, then it should obviously have been mentioned in the consent form; doing so would have made the defense of the case substantially easier.

In any event, on arrival at the teaching hospital, the admitting diagnosis was "injured left ureter." If this had

continued to be the reference throughout the hospitalization for the next three weeks, there probably would not
have been a medical malpractice case. As I mentioned, the
entries in the record from that point forward were by residents and other physicians in training. The entries, however, included the following:

- "Transected" ureter
- "Lacerated" ureter
- "Nicked" ureter
- "Cut" ureter
- "Traumatically injured" ureter
- Multiple references, of course, to "injured"
  ureter

A discharge summary was dictated by a junior resident who
was not involved in the surgical procedure. Instead, he was
dictating the note for the more senior resident who had
actually performed the operation where they removed this
patient's kidney to alleviate the problem of leaking urine.
The patient had rejected more complicated reconstructive
surgery of the ureter, and the surgery performed was a
nephrectomy, or removal, of her kidney. The discharge summary incorrectly made reference to a radiologic study,
describing it as a "retrograde nephrostogram." The study
was actually an antegrade nephrostogram, but more importantly, the resident indicated that it confirmed the transected ureter. If one looked carefully at the handwritten
note of the interventional radiologist, there was never a
mention of the word *transected* or *cut* or any other perjora-
tive term.

Because all of these references were made when there was no litigation, they were very difficult to rebut. The plaintiff's expert was relying on these notations made in a hospital with an excellent regional reputation.

House officers, students, and any physician making entries in hospital records should be wary of the consequences of their documentation. Often, junior people make entries in a record, everyone seems to repeat that entry, and it becomes the theme of a medical malpractice case even if unsupported by the actual medical evidence. Please be careful and be accurate, because you may be making life difficult for a colleague.

In this particular case we, happily, were able to prevail, in large part due to the fact that the surgeons did an excellent job on their own behalf at the time of trial, in spite of the trauma of going through that process. We also had excellent experts, including a reconstructive urologist who had done ureter surgery for years, who testified that the nephrostogram that we had reproduced and enlarged for jury viewing supported the proposition that the problem was a vascular injury resulting in ischemia to the ureter, leading to its tapering to the point of disruption, which was not consistent with a cut or transection.

None of the doctors at the teaching hospital had ever seen the area of injury to the ureter except in this radiologic study. When the kidney was removed, there was no exploration to examine the injured area of the ureter, nor am I suggesting that there should have been. The pathologic specimen consisted of the kidney and just the area of the ureter above where they had surgically cut it to remove the kidney. The point is that no one had seen the ureter. The X-ray study was the closest that anyone had come to seeing what had actually happened to the ureter, yet all of these house officers had created considerable confusion for the two defendants in the case.

Patient Transfers

Another recurring problem with record entries by junior staff occurs when patients are transferred from a hospital to a tertiary care center. We have had numbers of cases where an ambulance is sent out from a major hospital to an outlying community hospital to transport a newborn. I am sure that it's a very stressful situation for all concerned, but the transport team generally would consist of a nurse and an obstetrical or pediatric resident. Often, the transfer team makes an entry that the diagnosis is hypoxic ischemic encephalopathy (HIE). As it turns out in a later lawsuit, that diagnosis becomes the whole issue of the case: Did this infant actually suffer from hypoxia during the course of labor and delivery? We are confronted with the transfer note, which becomes the admitting diagnosis, generally made by another junior resident, and stays in the medical record.

Often, transfer teams gratuitously make comments about the fetal heart tracing, having had a very brief opportunity to look at one section of the tracing, and comment that there were "late decelerations" or generally that the tracing was "not reassuring of fetal well-being." Three years later, when the case is being reviewed by true experts in electronic fetal heart monitoring and they tell us that the tracing is per-

fectly reasonable, we have to overcome all of these earlier
inaccuracies.

Be careful. Be accurate. Recognize your own limitations
and level of training.

HOSPITALISTS

A relatively recent addition to the healthcare force is the
hospitalist. Generally speaking, these individuals are medical doctors or doctors of osteopathic medicine and, in some
cases, physician assistants or nurse practitioners who focus
on practicing in the inpatient setting. We will probably see,
in the very near future, fellowship programs and board cer-
tification for the hospitalist as a specialist. Presently, this
area seems to attract younger physicians and some foreign
medical graduates who feel that their training makes them
better suited to work in the inpatient setting and who find
the inpatient setting more interesting than an ambulatory
practice. Also, as a hospitalist, the physician does not have
to wait to establish a practice with a large roster of patients,
nor does she have to join an established group practice.
Generally, hospitalists are employed by hospitals, but some
large group practices hire their own hospitalists to cover
their own group of patients when they are hospitalized.

Advantages of Using Hospitalists

Part of the rationale behind the shift to the use of hospitalists was the gradual decrease in hours worked by residents,
as well as the valid complaints of primary care physicians

that they did not have adequate time to see people in the ambulatory setting. The use of hospitalists should free up some time of the busy primary care physician in that they will not be expected to make hospital rounds. With this time, they can see more patients or, even better, spend more time with the same number of patients.

Disadvantages of Using Hospitalists

The downside is that if you have a long-term relationship with a patient who is then hospitalized, particularly if it is for some period of time, the patient may be very disappointed or even upset that he doesn't receive a visit from his primary care physician. When recommending someone for hospital admission, it would be wise to explain gently the role of the hospitalist and why it is good for their safety and well-being that someone who is a fully accredited physician will be available 24 hours a day. The patient should also know that there will be continuity of care; the hospitalist will keep you advised of the patient's progress and consult with you regarding discharge plans and appropriate follow-up. You need to be certain that you provide adequate history and information of the problem requiring admission to the hospital so that the hospitalist has adequate data to follow your patient through that admission process.

Primary care physicians have, for years, felt reasonably comfortable in referring their patients to emergency rooms, and I think that using hospitalists is analogous to that situation. The hospitalist is another qualified physician, probably with a different mix of training but mostly internal medicine, who practices at a particular site (i.e., the hospital).

Again, make it clear to your patients what this individual's role will be. For years, when families have visited a patient in the hospital, the first question has been "Was the doctor in today?" They need to be educated that the doctor may not be the one they are accustomed to seeing but rather someone who only operates in the inpatient setting.

If you have a patient of long standing with a complicated medical history, and she is admitted directly from your practice to a hospital, where your understanding is that she will be seen by a hospitalist and that you will not be following her, you must take extra precautions that a full, complete, and detailed history is provided to the hospitalist on admission so that it will be part of the patient's permanent records. I see too many opportunities for errors in a handoff from a primary care physician to a hospitalist who has never had any involvement with the patient.

I saw a recent advertisement in the *New England Journal of Medicine* for a "nocturnist." I assume that this would be a hospitalist willing to work exclusively on the nightshift. I must say, I have not as yet had the privilege of defending a "nocturnist," but I anticipate that we might have some problems obtaining experts if we try to narrow it to nighttime practitioners to address the standard of care!

Two Examples: A Patient Transfer and a Shift Change

In two fairly recent situations we have been called upon to defend someone practicing as a hospitalist. In one case, a young woman came to the emergency room with a question of a stroke. The emergency room physician consulted with a neurologist who happened to be available very early in the morning. The neurologist saw the patient and decided that she was not a candidate for thrombolytic treatment, because the time of onset of her symptoms was unknown—she had awakened with the symptoms. The hospitalist was called shortly after she was seen by the neurologist to arrange for the admission workup.

The family of this patient requested a transfer to a major teaching hospital. Because the teaching hospital was on "diversion," it was unable to accept the patient in transfer until approximately eight hours later. The medical records from the teaching hospital later reflected that it had a very advanced investigational stroke service, and someone made a notation in the record that the patient might have been treated intra-arterially if seen sooner. The emergency room physician, the neurologist, and the hospitalist were all sued. The hospitalist was named for not arranging a more expeditious transfer, even though the institution requested by the family was on diversion, on the theory that he should have transferred her to another more sophisticated hospital or he should have made arrangements for her treatment at his hospital (which was not equipped to do this kind of treatment). In any event, after about nine months, and just as discovery in the case was beginning to develop, the plaintiff elected to voluntarily drop, or dismiss, the case.

The other recent case was a drug overdose, where the patient was taken to an emergency room about when shifts were changing. The only constant name that appeared in the record was that of the hospitalist, who was probably working a 12-hour shift at the time, thus crossing over the emergency room and the intensive care shift. As it turns out, the plaintiff sued every doctor whose name appeared in the record, including some who were not there. (We'll talk about this later in this chapter in the section on hospital records.) In any event, that case is still pending, and it would be inappropriate to discuss it further, except in the most general of terms.

Another Option to Relieve Physician Workload: Making Greater Use of Nurses

As an aside, since we were discussing how the use of hospitalists can help alleviate the burden on primary care physicians, a perspective appeared in the November 27, 2008, *New England Journal of Medicine* entitled "Staying One Step Ahead of Burnout." The article reports on efforts being made in the practice in question to make professional life more tolerable for primary care doctors. Obviously, such efforts will differ from third-party payer to third-party payer, but the article is well worth your attention. The subject practice makes extensive use of office nurses, who see to it that laboratory work is done prior to a visit so that it can be discussed at the visit, and they have a brief meeting with the doctor before the doctor goes into the examination room to discuss laboratory results from a prior visit and the results of the nurse's examination, including any current complaints. This workflow certainly makes for more efficient use of the physician's time and undoubtedly will lead to increased patient satisfaction, which directly contributes to fewer malpractice claims.

GROUP VISITS

A feature story ran in the *Boston Globe* of November 30, 2008, regarding the Harvard Vanguard Medical Associates's entitled *The Doctor Will See All of You Now* relative to so-called shared medical appointments. The report was also mentioned in the November 27, 2008, *New England Journal of Medicine.* Shared medical appointments are being employed on a trial basis at Harvard Vanguard. The story is about a cardiologist who saw nine patients in a group at a 4:00 PM session. Over the next 90 minutes, the cardiologist examined each patient in the presence of the group and discussed the patient's personal medical details, likewise in the presence of everyone. Apparently, patients are willing to sacrifice privacy for improved access to doctors. If a patient is willing to see the doctor in a group visit, she can get appointments sooner, and patients with similar problems and questions evidently feel that they can learn from one another during a group visit. If any part of the examination involves disrobing, the doctor and patient go to a private area for that portion of the visit.

Doctors evidently like group visits because they can increase their productivity without working more hours. It was reported that many insurers pay per patient what they would if these were individual visits, when a doctor might see only four to six patients in 90 minutes. Patient satisfaction was also reported as high, as the patients feel that they get to spend a lot more time with the physician and that hearing questions from other patients is helpful. Patients have to sign consent forms agreeing not to disclose information regarding any other patient, and if there are matters they don't wish to discuss with the group, they can speak privately with the physician at the end of the session. This experimental program, dealing with patients with similar problems, is a novel approach to the primary care physician shortage and problems with respect to time spent with patients, but it is fraught with unanswered questions:

- Does another patient really have an obligation to maintain confidentiality?
- Would another patient be liable if he violated the confidentiality of the information shared? There certainly is no regulatory or licensing board you could complain to for this kind of a breach of confidentiality.
- Will patients lose what little is left of the physician-patient relationship by not having one-on-one sessions with their providers?
- Will patients truly be willing to reveal concerns and problems in a group situation when they sometimes have difficulty doing so one on one?
- If advice is given about skipping or stopping a particular medication and one of the group has adverse consequences, will your defense end up with nine versions of what was said in a group meeting instead of one or two versions?
- I see from the article that the physician has an assistant take notes, but how are these notes monitored for individual accuracy and insertion in individual medical records?

- What is the chance that members of the group might know one another?

This is a newly developing program and is probably not for everyone. It should be done only in tightly monitored practice groups with sufficient personnel to ensure its smooth functioning for patient care and overall patient satisfaction. Many, many questions remain to be answered.

HOSPITAL RECORDS

It is difficult to know where to begin to talk about the problems generated by hospital records.

Missing Records

One of the most damaging situations involves missing records, particularly when the missing records are pertinent to the subject of a claim. Imagine yourself as the lawyer for a family who has questions about whether or not their infant may have suffered an injury in the labor and delivery process. You send a request with appropriate authorizations to the hospital, and you receive the records but no fetal heart tracings. After further investigation with the hospital, it tells you that staff cannot find those records; they have either gone to storage, been misfiled, or are just plain missing. That not only would raise your suspicions as a lawyer that something untoward had happened during the labor and delivery, but legally, it may create a presumption that because the hospital lost the records, those records would have been harmful to the defense.

Frequently, portions of records, which are the essence of a complaint by a patient, end up disappearing. I suspect that one of the mechanisms is that parts of the record are taken to a departmental or administrative meeting or hearing, or even a disciplinary hearing of an employee, and then they never make it back to the record. If an original record absolutely must be taken from the Medical Record Department, a full and complete copy should be inserted in its place with a notation that it is a copy, the date it was copied, and the person to whom the record was released. The least you can do if someone raises a complaint (not a lawsuit) about something that happened on your watch is respond by referring to the record. It is devastating to you as a healthcare provider when records are lost.

Fetal Heart Tracings

Fetal heart tracings have always been a problem. Most institutions that I have seen have never kept them with the patient's medical record, either the mother's record or that of the baby. They always seem to end up in a box somewhere with other fetal heart tracings to be sent off to storage. We have had cases where the hospital's storage area was flooded, damaging all of the fetal heart tracings beyond recognition, or they were not in the storage box when retrieved and had probably been misfiled.

We had one very serious labor and delivery case with a profoundly damaged child, and hospital staff were having an awful time trying to find the fetal heart tracings. There had been an extensive departmental review of both the nursing and obstetrical roles in the care of the mother during the course of a difficult labor and delivery, so we knew the tracings had been available for peer review. The minutes of the peer review meetings documented that the fetal heart tracings were supportive of fetal well-being; those tracings were at the meetings. I tried something novel and requested that the Department of Obstetrics and Gynecology post a reward consisting of free pizzas for members of the department for a month. Within a week, the fetal heart tracings appeared, after having been found in an unmarked cardboard box in the department's conference room. With the advent of digital and electronic records, records should not go missing as frequently—with just a caveat or two. We have finally learned, through a company that does visual aids for defense firms in our area, how to have the original fetal heart tracings (if they can be found), complete with nurses notes, scanned so that expert reviewers can look at the tracings in real time and in color. It made the review process much more meaningful, and we were able to transfer that technology to an actual courtroom where instead of showing piles of paper, we showed the most accurate possible reproduction of the tracing to a jury.

We recently tried to obtain a fetal monitor tracing from one of the hospitals that we represent. We received the standard printed copies of the tracing, which often are cut off so that you miss blocks of time on the tracing and have to go back and get more copies and then piece them together. We made a request for a "live, real-time" copy and were told that the hospital's technology did not permit staff to make a CD or DVD from the database. If you are an obstetrician or an administrator, you should at least look into the technological options available to preserve these studies so that they can be used in an effective manner.

Example: Obstetrical Records

Let me point out another potential problem, which has likewise been around for years but may be complicated further by HIPAA or people's overreading of HIPAA. We had a case where a young woman was seen at an outlying hospital and had a biophysical profile, which was relatively normal but showed a fetal heart tracing that was not reassuring of the welfare of the fetus. Because this was an immature fetus, the community hospital transferred the patient to a teaching institution. The patient was transferred with copies (although I suspect some of the pages were originals) of the transferring hospital's records with her in the ambulance. Obviously, the clinicians at the second facility referred to these in evaluating this patient. The biophysical profile was repeated, and it was essentially the same as at the outlying hospital. The obstetrical team tried to assess the well-being of the fetus, including calling for cardiac evaluations to make sure that, before intervening, they would have a reasonably healthy baby. A few hours later, the tracing was worse, and they proceeded to a cesarean section. The child survived for about a day.

We requested a copy of the record from the outlying hospital and received it, but it did not include the biophysical profile or a physical evaluation of the mother. These records were clearly missing. We did several subpoenas to the Medical Records Department, including one requesting the personal presence of the head of the department.

I then went with the claim representative to the hospital where our clients were employed and asked to have a look at the original record. In the original record, in a pocket labeled "correspondence," were copies of all of the records from the outlying hospital. I made copies of those, sent them to the outlying hospital, and asked why they had not been included in the records that we had subpoenaed. The response was that "they had been converting to electronic records and some of their records were out being scanned and they must have been misplaced."

I then asked our clients' hospital why we had not been furnished these records, since they obviously were part of the care and treatment of the woman at the teaching facility. I was told by the Medical Records Department that these were records of another institution and I would have to get them from that institution. That is all well and good, provided that the other institution knows how to find its own records.

We got this response even though we had served a subpoena, which included a request, as we do in all cases, for any records of other hospitals or referring physicians and correspondence that are part of the documentation within the record. One other record that had been part of the referring hospital's paperwork was the prenatal records from an obstetrical clinic. The hospital had these records but told me that they were from "another provider" and would not be produced. It has always been my understanding that at a certain time in a pregnancy, the obstetrical provider sends the prenatal records to the hospital or clinic where she expects the patient to deliver. Why these are not considered part of hospital records by certain medical record directors is beyond me. Those of you out there who have anything to do with medical records, administratively or even as a clinician, should check your own affiliated hospitals to find out what their policies are with regard to what is kept in a record and what is available should someone request copies. It doesn't help you if appropriate requests for records are met with incomplete records.

Example: A "Broken" Neck

Let me touch on one more hospital record case. In a recent case that was tried before an arbitrator and resulted in a finding in favor of a nurse midwife and an obstetrician, the central issue was whether during the course of a difficult delivery involving shoulder dystocia, the defendants, and particularly the nurse midwife, had used excessive force, resulting in fracturing the neck of the fetus and the infant's death. The whole scenario arose primarily because of miscommunication and, later, systemic problems, which made it very difficult to convince the unfortunate parents that the care providers had done nothing wrong.

The parents of this baby were non-English speaking, and after the incident, they met with patient representatives and some members of the treatment team. Members of the treatment team were called away frequently, so there was no real continuity to the meeting. (In fact, one of the meetings with the family was called on September 11, 2001; the events of that day justifiably resulted in a breakup of the meeting. Talk about bad things happening!) In any event, the body of the newborn had been sent to a nearby teaching hospital affiliated with the delivery hospital for purposes of an autopsy. Whether something was lost in translation or not, the family had requested that the autopsy be limited to the head and neck, because they were present at the labor and delivery and observed that complications had occurred. After the body had been delivered to the teaching hospital, the staff there performed imaging studies, which revealed "no fracture" or "breaks" but did show some "soft tissue injury" to the neck. At a subsequent meeting with the parents and after misunderstandings, misinterpretations, and translations, the parents came away with the impression that "the baby's neck had been broken." This became the theme of the entire case. Incredibly, in spite of many efforts, we were unable to obtain the X-rays done at the hospital where the autopsy had been performed. The Pathology Department at that hospital told us that it did not keep X-rays. The X-ray department said that it had no way of tracking X-rays—it had no patient number, since the mother had never been a patient at the institution where the autopsy had been performed and the baby was only there for an autopsy.

This situation could have been avoided simply by a mechanism that permitted the tracking of X-rays. For example, the hospital that referred the case for autopsy had a contractual arrangement with the teaching hospital to perform autopsies on stillborns and postnatal deaths. There should have been a procedural requirement that any X-rays or lab work done by the teaching hospital be returned to the hospital where the incident occurred.

Fortunately, the arbitrator believed that both the certified nurse midwife and the obstetrician complied with the standard of care and issued a binding finding in their behalf.

Complete Records Promptly

Records also need to be completed in a timely fashion. While a licensing board may not go after you for not completing records on time, I can assure you that plaintiffs' lawyers will. Sometimes they have a copy of the record before you even dictate an operative report or, in some cases, a discharge summary. While the delay may be perfectly innocent, jurors often wonder why so much time went by before you completed dictation. An operative note, for example, that is dictated a week or two after a patient has surgical complications requiring transfer to another institution tends to appear self-protective. The best dictation of a procedure is done immediately afterward. It is also a good idea to read the transcription.

Records Should Be Clear and Thorough

Although shoddy medical records, in and of themselves, are not a cause of liability, they certainly put you at a distinct disadvantage. You need to be able to answer questions from a patient, first to avoid a claim and, later should a claim arise, as to the evidence supporting your course of treatment. If you don't have those records or they are imprecise, then you have only your recollections or your comments to a fact finder that "this is my customary and usual practice," as supporting your standard of care. Such evidence can be quite shaky. In and of itself, a jury could consider the lack of documentation to be poor practice or even questionable judgment.

Medical records should show clearly what you did for a patient and the manner in which it was done, and they should be readily understandable by the average member of the profession. A record should show upon its face that nothing was neglected and that the physician met the standard of care demanded by the law. A good medical record should also show a patient's lack of compliance or minimal compliance with your recommendations and instructions, if applicable. Any letters sent to the patient or other providers should be kept as part of the record. Try not to use ambiguous statements or comments, which will be interpreted as an inference of negligence on your part; examples include *inadvertently* and *iatrogenic* (all plaintiff lawyers know that these words mean a medical error). The date and time of every entry should be noted. We look at records all the time that have the day and month but not the year recorded, and when you are looking at records two, three, or five years down the road, their date is by no means evident.

Comments in the record should include how the patient re-sponded to treatment and whether the patient is following the prescribed plan of care. Notations should be made of discussions you have with any other physician, even if as a so-called "curbside consult." When you make an entry in the record, particularly in the hospital setting, try to include facts, not just conclusions. If the patient falls, for example, on the way to the bathroom, the records should include a direct quote from the patient that she lost her balance and fell rather than your conclusion that "patient apparently fell." Please do not include in the record the fact that an incident report has been filed. These are indications of a triggering event leading to peer review. To include that information piques the curiosity of a potential claimant who looks at the medical record. The fact that, in most cases, we can prevent the introduction into evidence of the content of the incident report or peer review doesn't really erase the presence of the entry, sitting in the minds of the jury and suggesting something untoward.

If you are deviating from recommended dosages for a particular patient, please be careful to document your reasons for the deviation and issue orders to monitor the patient carefully for potential side effects and reactions. Drugs are prescribed every day outside of the limits of the PDR, which is really published to protect drug manufacturers, but to protect yourself, you need to document why you have done something that may not be in strict compliance with the PDR or other guidelines.

Sample Medical Record Entries

To lighten things up a bit, I must say that over the years, I have collected a number of rather bizarre entries in medical records. A sampling follows:

- Patient's medical history has been remarkable with only a 40-pound weight gain in the past three days.
- Patient had waffles for breakfast and anorexia for lunch.
- Patient has two teenage children, but no other abnormalities.
- Between you and me, we ought to be able to get this lady pregnant.

- The patient was to have a bowel resection. However, he took a job as a stockbroker instead.
- Healthy appearing, decrepit 69-year-old male, mentally alert but forgetful.
- Discharge status: Alive, but without my permission.
- The patient has been depressed since she began seeing me in 1993.
- She stated that she had been constipated for most of her life, until she got a divorce.

Obviously, lawyers are experts at saying rather outrageous things that may not be transcription errors, such as asking the following questions (Please note that these are not transcription errors):

Attorney: This myasthenia gravis, does it affect your memory at all?
Witness: Yes.
Attorney: And in what ways does it affect your memory?
Witness: I forget.
Attorney: You forgot? Can you give us an example of something you forgot?

Attorney: Now doctor, isn't it true that when a person dies in his sleep, he doesn't know about it until the next morning?
Witness: Did you actually pass the bar exam?

Attorney: The youngest son, the 20-year-old, how old is he?
Witness: Uh, he's 20.

Attorney: How was your first marriage terminated?
Witness: By death.
Attorney: And by whose death was it terminated?
Witness: Now whose death do you suppose terminated it?

Attorney: Doctor, how many of your autopsies have you performed on dead people?
Witness: All my autopsies are performed on dead people. Would you like to rephrase that?[1]

Correction of Errors

Many errors in transcription either go unrecognized or are simply scratched through by the physician, giving an impression of diminished attention or even carelessness. There may be some "stock" descriptions of certain procedures. However, I can assure you, having seen this, that it is not helpful to either defending a claim or preventing a claim when you have a multipage procedure note that is dictated and transcribed six months after a procedure, when a reasonable physician could not possibly remember the technical details of how a procedure was performed in such minute detail.

[1] "Disorder in the Court." Sevilla, W. W. Norton, 1999.

Another fairly recent case, which went to trial, involved two orthopedic surgeons and a registered nurse. The patient had had his second knee replacement done by Surgeon Number One. On postoperative day three, the house staff felt that the patient had a postoperative ileus. A flat-plate abdominal film was taken and interpreted by the radiologist as showing possible Ogilvy's syndrome, which involves a large collection of air in the colon. If not decompressed, the air can lead to perforation. Perforation happened in this case, resulting in the patient's death. The orthopedic resident said that he telephoned the operating surgeon and told him of the X-ray results. The operating surgeon did not know what Ogilvy's syndrome was and could have saved a great deal of difficulty by calling the radiologist to find out.

In the early morning hours, the covering orthopedist was called to the patient's bedside because the patient had coffee-ground emesis. There was some delay in that surgeon getting to the hospital, and when he tried to intubate the patient, which he hadn't done for many years, the patient coded and expired. The covering physician was asked why he hadn't called for a surgical resident or someone else in the hospital to assist in intubation. He replied that it was hospital protocol that orthopedics could not directly ask a general surgery resident for assistance but had to go through a more senior attending general surgeon to initiate the referral process.

So far, we have seen in this example terrible communication errors. Better communication might have saved the patient and certainly would have saved a lawsuit. To top things off, the nurse failed to record the patient's vital signs at any time during his shift, although he claims that he took them at the appropriate intervals. This is why he ended up as a defendant. For whatever reason, a jury returned a verdict in favor of the two orthopedists and the nurse.

Let me repeat, never change records. If it is discovered that you changed or altered a record, except by following hospital procedure, your goose is cooked. The hospital procedure for changing a record should be that you draw a single line through the erroneous entry so that it can still be seen and you write "error" next to the corrected entry. Altering a record in any other way has the disastrous effect of making otherwise defensible cases big losers. The angrier a jury becomes with a healthcare provider, the higher the dollar amount of the verdict will be. Writing legibly is equally important in the in-hospital setting and in the office; electronic medical records will resolve the legibility problem, but there will always be some handwriting in records. You should also exercise vigilance in ensuring that entries in the electronic record are accurate.

Read Nurses' Notes

Please try to read nurse's notes. Let me give just a couple of examples of cases that required settlement because of the failure of a surgeon to read notes. I hear surgeons all the time say that they don't have time; instead, they get a brief oral report from the nurse before seeing the patient. The problem is that a written note from an earlier shift might not make it into the nurse's oral report, making this verbal exchange unreliable. We have had cases of postoperative infections where a physician has said that there was "nothing to culture." The problem was the nurse's notes reporting "drainage from wound" and, even after the note of "nothing to culture," a nurse's note of "wound continues to drain." Another case involved spinal surgery where the physical therapist note indicated "new postoperative radiating pain down the right leg." The physician never saw this note and discharged the patient to a rehabilitation hospital where similar notations were made. About two months postoperatively, when the patient complained to the surgeon, a CAT scan revealed a misplaced screw. This necessitated a second surgery, and the patient made a claim of permanent injury. Without the mix-up, the patient would still have needed a second surgery to back off the screw. However, had it been done while he was still an inpatient from the initial surgery, the chances of any long-term injury or disability would have been minimal, and there would have been no question about the standard of care.

Is Your Name on a Record It Shouldn't Be On?

Check periodically to see how your hospital(s) handle(s) addressographs. Let me give you a few examples.

In one case, a psychiatrist who had his private practice in a hospital-based office was generally the most available of the staff, at least physically. The practice was often to put the patient data and name of this psychiatrist as the attending physician, even though he was not going to be the attending physician the next day and, in fact, never had any encounters with the patient at all.

Regrettably, one day a patient escaped from the hospital and committed suicide, and the psychiatrist ended up being sued. The psychiatric staff operated in two teams. My client was part of Team II, and the assignments for attending coverage were rotated. Even though this patient was assigned to Team I and should have been the responsibility of a different psychiatrist, the record clearly indicated that my client was the "attending physician" and "admitting physician." The chief of the department testified at deposition and at trial that placing my client's name on the addressograph was purely an administrative process and in no way indicated that he was acting as the physician for that patient. Happily, the hospital discontinued the practice but not before a lengthy, very unpleasant trial, which fortunately was resolved in favor of my psychiatrist client.

We once defended a case where an obstetrical attending physician at a large maternity hospital had a stamp of her signature to use in cosigning notes of house staff. The requirement of the hospital was that all house officer notes be cosigned by an attending. The problem was that in practice, the more senior residents or the chief resident would often use the stamp, which was readily available, to keep the paperwork moving. We went through a trial defending this doctor, who was only in the case because of the rubber stamp on the record and who testified that she had never had any involvement with the patient. We actually brought in a few other women to sit near our client during the trial, and the patient and her husband were unable to identify her in the courtroom. The signature stamp is a practice to be avoided, and if you plan to use it, be certain that you are the only person who has access to a facsimile of your signature.

In another recent case, the patient was in the emergency room of the hospital for a drug overdose, and at about 4:00 PM, the decision was made to transfer her to the intensive care unit. She had been accepted but was waiting for a bed. One of the issues among the doctors when we first met with them was who "owned" this patient. The decision to transfer had occurred when shifts were changing, and the practice, regrettably, was that a ward clerk or someone in a secretarial position would stamp blank progress note sheets with the name of the attending who happened to be present in the intensive care unit (ICU). By the time the patient actually made it to the intensive care unit, that physician had gone home. The daytime ICU physician was assigned to sign electronically the history and physical exam done by the ICU resident who had examined the patient in the emergency department. The history and exam were not transcribed and, therefore, were not available for signature until the following day, approximately eight hours after the patient had expired. The same physician did not actually sign the history and physical for several days.

To further complicate the case, another ICU physician was sued who was not in the hospital on the evening in question. She was on beeper call for the group beginning in the early evening and claimed that she was only to be available for calls outside the ICU for patients with general pulmonary problems, since staff were always on duty in the ICU. The emergency room physician wrote in his note that he had a telephone discussion with this particular doctor and said, "Doctor Blank is comfortable with this." The emergency room doctor said that he had discussed the question of intubation with this doctor on the telephone and they had agreed not to intubate. The pulmonary physician said that she would not have addressed the question of intubation at all under these circumstances and would have told the emergency room physician to talk with the physician in the ICU about any patient who was headed there.

This situation was just a nightmare waiting to happen. Fortunately, the lawyer for the patient's family was fairly reasonable. We showed them documentation, and they agreed to dismiss the two ICU physicians who had no contact with the patient.

"Curbside" Consults

Informal consults, or what are sometimes referred to as *curbside* consults, come back to haunt people on a regular basis. We have had a number of cases where a treating physician has made a note saying that she has discussed the patient's case with a particular doctor. The discussion may have been in the hallway or by a quick telephone call. What happens is that, when the plaintiff's lawyer becomes aware that a consultation occurred with another physician, that physician ends up being added to the case. Of course, the consulted physician has absolutely no recollection of a brief conversation with a colleague that may have occurred two or three years earlier. Be very careful how you record these types of consults. If you feel compelled to mention in the note that you had an informal consult, call it that. You can even say, "We had a curbside consult." You may say, "I happened to see Doctor X in the cafeteria and mentioned this case, and he generally agreed with my plan of action." Don't put this other physician on the spot.

Workflow: Who's In Charge?

Another problem when reading a hospital record is trying to determine who was in charge. This is not only complicated when dealing with future legal problems with a patient, but it is reportedly an ongoing problem while patients are in the hospital. Many patients report that they never seem to be able to find out who is managing the traffic when it comes to their own or a loved one's healthcare. Residents are reluctant to call attendings. Many patients don't recognize the gradations in responsibility within a teaching hospital setting and sometimes never even get to speak with an attending physician. This situation needs to be corrected. If you are an attending physician in a training hospital, you need to have more personal contact with patients, even though they may be taken care of on a daily basis by resident physicians who are perfectly competent.

Patients need to know that someone is in charge. Where a major problem arises with a patient, a family knows endless frustration and anger when they can't find out whom they really need to talk with to get some resolution. This is a hot bed for potential medical malpractice claims. You would be well served to make it clear to your resident physicians that they need to contact you on a regular basis and not be concerned that you will think that they don't know what they are doing or that they lack expertise. In many cases I have seen, residents felt that they should not contact an attending physician because the attending would think that they are "bothering them" or "they don't know what they are doing." This whole atmosphere needs to be modified. You need to be an active participant in the team process of caring for patients in the teaching hospital setting. Doing so will not only provide better care but will help reduce claims against you individually.

IMAGING

When using the term *X-rays* in this section, I mean to include all forms of imaging studies.

Missing Images

A recurring problem, which we hope will be eliminated by the use of digital studies, has been the rather casual practice of handing over original films to patients, patient attorneys, or other treaters. Often, when we receive a notice of a claim, no X-rays are available in the radiology department, and sometimes there is no record of where they went. Only through repeated requests to the attorneys for the patient do we finally end up "borrowing" X-rays, which technically are the property of the hospital or physician's office where the studies were done. It can often take us months and months to obtain original films—a very frustrating process, particularly when we are trying to set up initial meetings with radiology defendants.

If you still use films, the practice should be not to give original X-rays to the patient. If a clinician contacts you saying that he absolutely must have the original study to treat the patient, then the image can be transferred but with careful documentation: a notation that the images are to be returned within 30 days and a tickler system follow-up to obtain the return of the films. It is also not in the interest of good patient care for a radiologist to look at current films and make a notation "prior films not available for comparison." It's not that unusual for a patient to pick up films for review by an attorney while continuing her medical treatment at the institution where the films were taken. It's awkward when they are still missing a year or two later.

Markings on Films

This is another nightmare for defense counsel and defendants in malpractice cases. It occurs most frequently in mammography, but we have seen it in all types of imaging studies. Often, when a diagnosis is made, "someone," whether it be a surgeon or a subsequent radiologist, looks at a prior study and then marks off the questionable lesion that they now, in retrospect, can see on a new film or CT scan. It's like having arrows saying, "Here's a potential malpractice claim."

Frequently, these original films, as I have indicated, wind up in the possession of the plaintiff. It is not fair to have films with markings reviewed by an expert for the plaintiff who now obviously knows immediately where the questionable area is. You will never find a case where a plaintiff attorney has removed these wax markings, which are meant to be neither diagnostic nor even particularly accurate with respect to the exact location and dimensions of a particular lesion, before sending the films to an expert. We have appeared before judges a number of times to request permission to remove these markings from the original films to have an expert review them fairly with as prospective a perspective as possible when knowing that the patient had a problem. Most judges say that they will not "alter" or "tamper with" the evidence in a case. Only a very sophisticated trial judge will recognize how basically unfair it is to a defendant to have the films reviewed in that condition. In those cases, we have had copies made showing where the marks are; the marks are then removed for review by experts (we always make copies of the originals without the markings); and the films are returned to the plaintiff's attorney, who can feel free to put the marks back where they were as shown on the copy. In that case, we still deal with the issue of which film will be used at the time of trial.

It is bad enough that we deal with known retrospective bias in reviewing imaging studies without having directional signs placed by, sometimes, our client and, more often, by a colleague. What to do? If the markings are truly needed in the care and treatment of a patient, make a copy and put the markings on the copy for a subsequent treater. If the markings are placed on the film, there again should be some kind of follow-up tickler so that when you learn that the treatment is complete, these markings can be removed. They are not part of the patient's treatment and are not intended as such.

Requisition Forms

Often in breast cancer cases, a dispute arises as to whether the patient reported that she had discovered a lump on self-examination, and the requisition form is missing. It generally does not become part of the traditional hospital record but is either kept within the X-ray "jacket" or is noted on the X-ray jacket or folder itself. For whatever reason, these forms tend to go astray, and there needs to be a way to protect yourself.

Once, in a case where we were defending a radiologist, a primary care physician testified that she was not aware of the difference between a screening and a diagnostic mammogram. She had actually felt the lump in the patient's breast, which she did not feel was significant, and just told her that she should go for a screening mammogram. At the institution in question, women could self-refer for mammography. This patient showed up with no paperwork whatsoever, and the requisition form or information made out by the technician was missing in action. This patient was a young woman in her 40s who later, at the time of diagnosis, had stage IV breast cancer. The radiologist, obviously, would have conducted a different kind of study had the clinician either reported the lump, sent a requisition herself, or ordered a diagnostic—rather than screening—mammogram.

How can these situations be avoided? You need to have some safeguard procedures in place, such as the following:

- A nurse practitioner or physician's assistant conducts a breast examination prior to a planned screening mammogram.
- Since the radiologist is not often present, requisition forms with the patient's clinical data, which should be very brief, should be attached to one of the films that's placed for

viewing by the radiologist (any kind of alternative safety procedure would be satisfactory).

- With digital mammography, will it be possible for you to indicate in your dictation the degrees of magnification and views that you used or any enhancements so that in the future we'd be able to reproduce accurately the conditions under which you reviewed the film and what the film most accurately looked like? (I don't pretend to know the answer to this one.)
- The average woman, when she receives a postcard that her mammogram was "negative" or "normal" or "unchanged," feels that the mammogram has ruled out any reasonable likelihood of her having breast cancer. Whatever the underlying error rate is in mammography, whether it be 10 percent or 15 percent, patients should be made aware of it so that they do not come away with the mistaken impression that something should have been seen when a year or two later a diagnosis is made. Again, perception is really critical to the mind-set of the average patient in contemplating whether to bring a claim. You have to remember that in radiology cases, the patients have not had any direct contact with the radiologist. Therefore, the normal, warm, trusting relationship, which often prevents potential errors from becoming real claims, has no chance to develop.

Retrospective Bias

While we are discussing radiologists, I would like to explore the concept of "retrospective bias." This is a well-recognized phenomenon in radiology, and a number of articles have been written on the subject. Some of the articles have made reference to the old children's picture puzzle called "Where's Waldo." Someone who is trying to solve the Where's Waldo puzzle knows ahead of time that Waldo is in the picture puzzle yet still has a great deal of difficulty finding him. Once you can see Waldo, however, it's easy, and you can't believe that you didn't pick it up right away. The situation for a radiologist in looking at a film is that he doesn't even know if there *is* a Waldo in the picture, yet the radiologist is expected during a lawsuit three or four years down the road to have known what was lurking in these black and white and gray shades of contrast.

Often, my own client will tell me that as soon as she looks at the films after being notified of the lawsuit, she could see the area in question. How does this affect the radiologist's liability? We recently conducted a focus group with a jury of 12 whom we selected based on what we felt would be the average composition of a jury in the county in which a lung cancer case was expected to be tried. The defendant radiologist had testified at his deposition that "in retrospect," he could see the lesion in question. Our expert reviewers, knowing when they did the review that they were looking at a film showing a potential problem (a luxury that the interpreting radiologist did not have), felt that the reasonable radiologist would not have made the diagnosis "prospectively." We wanted to test how a potential jury would feel about a case where the doctor could see a problem, lesion, or nodule retrospectively. Interestingly, the 12 jurors split evenly. Six jurors felt that they, as laypeople, could see the area in question. So much for expertise! These same six jurors also felt that, if the doctor could see it in retrospect, that was similar to an admission that he should have seen it at the outset. The other six jurors grasped the subtle concept and felt that a radiologist could not have been expected to have picked this up and reported it at the time that he was reviewing the films.

This is a very difficult area for radiologists, lawyers, and even jurors to deal with. Some years ago, a very prominent mammographer told me that I would have big trouble if my client could see something in retrospect, because people would think that he should have seen it at the time of the examination. On the other hand, one has to be truthful, and if you can see it with the benefit of the "retrospectro-scope," then you cannot be untruthful to yourself or to the process. Please be careful how you report when you are dictating regarding prior films. It is very problematic when in your dictated report, you say that "in retrospect" a 0.8 centimeter lesion is seen in the area in question. This really almost seals the fate of a potential radiology defendant in a later case. I would recommend that you leave retrospectives out of your dictated reports.

Second Readers of Images

At a number of institutions and practices, certain studies, particularly mammography, have second readers. Some-times it's difficult to tell from a record who did the first read, who did the second read, and when. I have certainly had a number of cases where radiologists have spent a lot of time explaining the procedure and what happens when there may be some disagreement. Is there a read and then a dictation? Is the second reader merely reviewing the film, or does that person correct the dictation? In any event, when the final product is produced, does anyone know who truly completed the interpretation for purposes of treatment of the patient?

We have had several cases where both readers have been sued in a case, and in a few cases dealing with mammography, the plaintiffs sued radiologists who had interpreted films over a three- or four-year period. We ended up with seven or eight mammographers as defendants, because as chance would have it, they were back and forth doing second reads for one another. The only potential benefit of this process is that juries tend to believe so many radiologists could not be wrong. I think that juries deal basically in a fair manner with physician defendants, and if two, three, or four radiologists have made similar or the same interpretations of films, it is difficult for them to substitute their own judgment based on the expert testimony of a "hired gun" at the time of trial.

Record Magnification, Views, and So Forth

We are already seeing some cases involving digital mammography where this is an issue. Plaintiff lawyers, who can be very imaginative, will take the digital study and actually do a PowerPoint presentation. With the benefit of hindsight, it's very effective for a plaintiff to zoom in on an area that later turns out to be a malignant lesion. The practical problem that we have is that it's difficult, if not impossible, to know exactly how the radiologist viewed the study. What were the degrees of magnification? I always ask radiologists what the degree of magnification is of their handheld magnifiers, and I'm always surprised that most doctors have no idea. Not a good answer to a plaintiff lawyer. What views, what contrasts, etc. were employed in arriving at the diagnosis? If there are standard ways of looking at digital studies, that is fine, but if you deviate from standard practice to look at the mammogram in some different way, you should indicate that in your report. Otherwise, it will be practically impossible to re-create how you viewed the images. It's easy for a plaintiff's expert, in retrospect, to say the tumor would have been seen on a particular view or with more or less contrast and because there was a questionable area, you should have used these additional techniques.

Radiology Reports
You must provide sufficient information to the clinician to alert him to any potential problems with the patient. You cannot always rely on the level of astuteness of the referring physician when you dictate your report.

For example, we have a case of multiple myeloma where the primary issue is whether the physician who interpreted the CT scan gave adequate information to the primary care physician. The comment by the radiologist was "diffuse heterogeneous bone marrow" When I first met with my client, he said that he should have reported that a neoplastic process might have been occurring and that further clinical follow-up was required. I felt, on the other hand, that the referring physician, if he didn't understand the report, should have called the radiologist to find out what he was talking about. In any event, what happened was that the referring physician ordered a bone density exam in his office, which, of course, is notoriously inaccurate for multiple myeloma but indicated that he had read the CT report.

The other problem in this case—which comes back to one of the other major problems in malpractice cases, communication—is that the patient went from the primary care doctor to my client for the CT, then off to a consult at a second hospital who ordered a bone scan. Bone scan examinations are likewise inaccurate for multiple myeloma. The bone scan radiologist at a different hospital did notice a certain degree of uptake, which might have been consistent with an old traumatic injury. He naturally was unaware of any of the earlier studies, ordered a plain chest film that day, and interpreted that as showing old trauma. We are defending both radiologists, and the consult is also a defendant. Interestingly, the patient had a wonderful relationship with the primary care physician, who really was the problem in that he was not directing traffic in an appropriate manner. Sending the patient to different institutions for different studies, then not coordinating this process and not having these expert evaluators aware of what had happened at other institutions, was the error that led to this malpractice case—but not against the primary care physician because of an excellent physician-patient relationship.

When you are managing the care of a patient, coordinate care. It is incredible that you would send someone to different institutions for different studies at the same time that you were trying to evaluate the patient for the same condition. How you would expect a rational evaluation of all of the evidence with respect to your patient is beyond me. Now I recognize that the process depends on what part of the country you are in and how many institutions are available to you, but in areas where there are multiple institutions, it is not a good idea to move people around so much.

Technological Advances

Radiology has, of course, advanced to such incredible degrees where radiologists do 3D studies and interventional procedures that were beyond the imagination of the average layperson and even physicians only a decade or so ago. These advances mean that you need to be even more cautious in the expectations you leave with the patient of a particular study or procedure. It is really beyond the scope of this book to talk about all of the advances in medicine or even just within radiology, except to note that they are incredible and almost universally beneficial to the welfare of patients. With each of these advances, however, come risks. Diligence in keeping patients informed of potential complications and risks with advanced procedures should be ever on your mind to avoid unpleasantness.

Equipment Malfunction

You should periodically check the condition of the medical equipment that you use. Document any deficiencies in medical equipment, because I assure you that the medical equipment manufacturers will defend vigorously any claim that their equipment might have contributed to a mishap. While the institution may be responsible for reporting medical equipment errors and problems under the medical safety laws, you are the individual who can be most affected. Therefore, you should take careful measures to ensure that any equipment that may have malfunctioned is preserved and even checked by experts prior to being turned over to the manufacturer or governmental agency, because you will never see it again. Think of an equipment malfunction as an event that should have good medical documentation, just like any other adverse incident that could occur.

THE "DIFFICULT" PHYSICIAN

Whatever you do in your career, try not to be a "difficult" provider. You not only make the people around you miserable, but it will absolutely come back to bite you on the tail. I have had the privilege of meeting and working with some of the outstanding physicians in the country, and the truly great physicians that I have encountered were always humble, friendly, and admired by their office and hospital staff. The problem provider does not enjoy that kind of rapport with those about him. Why it happens, I do not really know but will leave it to others within the profession to come up with a diagnosis. What I can tell you is that anger and control problems will come back to haunt you.

We have had a number of cases involving surgeons who left the operating room during a procedure. Some of the cases ended up as medical malpractice cases, and others ended up as disciplinary proceedings before medical boards. In most of the cases, the physician's absence caused no harm. Historically, attending surgeons have remained in the operating room during the major parts of surgical procedures. Under Medicare, documentation must certify that they were present for the major parts of a procedure. However, it is medically appropriate for a surgeon to leave the closing of surgical wounds to an experienced chief resident or senior resident and to go about her business; otherwise, surgeons would never be able to get a reasonable number of cases accomplished in a given day.

So why does leaving the operating room sometimes result in a lawsuit or disciplinary hearing? In each of the cases that I have seen, when a physician has left the operating room and doing so involved even a slight deviation from hospital protocols, the surgeon has been reported to administration by staff to whom they have been obnoxious for a long time. You must understand that your conduct toward others does not go unnoticed. Interestingly, these are cases where the public reaction is one of disbelief and shock that the surgeon in whom they placed so much faith and trust had actually walked out on a case before its completion.

In these litigious days, it might be wise to tell patients that you have multiple cases on a particular day, that you are always present to do any and all of the complicated parts of the case, and that your assistants will do very routine matters other than assisting you. I recognize that disclosing this information is not general procedure in most surgical practices, but it would be helpful in keeping you out of a lawsuit and/or disciplinary proceedings.

Ranting, raving, and throwing things at people not only reflects questionable stability and lack of maturity but will lead to major problems as you go through your professional life. We have seen a number of cases of physicians who were involved in several malpractice cases, and when we looked carefully at their credentials files, they had been referred for anger management and other intervention programs. Try to consider how your conduct affects those around you and be constructive instead of engaging in destructive behavior, which in the long run will only harm you. If a resident, physician's assistant, technician, or other allied professional has attitude problems, he is generally dealt with rapidly and constructively. Don't think that you are any different; try to accept suggestions of colleagues and administrators to improve your professional life.

I have been tempted to withdraw from one or two cases because of my inability to get along with my own client. I was told by at least one client that he did not need to meet with me to prepare for a case, because he spent substantial time lecturing physicians and providers in continuing medical education programs and couldn't possibly learn anything from me. I told him that it would be malpractice on my part not to meet with him or to prepare him for trial. We finally did meet, and he didn't like the way I was going to ask a particular series of questions at the trial. I invited him to tell me how he would like the questions phrased. He did so. I wrote them down and told him that I would ask him exactly those questions at the time of trial, but I was interested in how he would respond. He gave me very reasonable explanations in response to his own questions. During the course of the trial, however, when I asked those very same questions, he stared blankly at me and asked me, "Could you repeat the question?" I was frankly a bit perturbed and replied, "Let me repeat it, and if you don't understand it this time, then we are both in trouble." I repeated his exact question and he genuinely bobbled the answer. In any event, it was a wrongful death case that proceeded through trial. Toward the end of the case, the doctor told me that he was going to present his own final argument to the jury, and we had a heated exchange of words in the courthouse lobby, ending by my presenting the closing argument.

At the end of the case, the jury found in favor of both my client and another physician defendant. My client had told me during the trial that there was a particular juror who, in his opinion, obviously liked him. I had an opportunity to speak with several of the jurors afterward, including this particular woman. She told me that if she ever woke up on a hospital stretcher and saw this doctor about to treat her, she would jump off the stretcher and run out the door. I asked her how she could have found in his favor, and she said that "I do not believe that anything that he did caused the death of this woman." Well, there's a juror who truly listened to what she was told by a judge and decided the case solely on the medical facts and opinions.

When I reported the favorable verdict to my client, he asked me if I had spoken with the jurors and particularly this one woman and wanted to know what she said. I told him that she said "she thought you were cute." I didn't think that it was going to be productive to get into any further discussion.

Those of you with this kind of attitude need to change. You certainly don't want to get into unnecessary trouble. You don't want to irritate people who have the obligation to protect you when you do get into trouble. And you will make your life much more pleasant.

Even as I write this, I am frustrated by my inability even to coordinate a meeting with two gynecologists who have been subpoenaed by a licensing board to testify in a case involving yet another healthcare provider. I was asked to represent both physicians by their insurer, so they are not expending any money on their own behalf. For whatever reason, one of the gynecologists refuses even to engage me in email or telephone discussions. When I send her an email and copy the claim representative of the hospital, she only responds to the claim representative and not to me. At least at this point, she is only a witness. With this kind of attitude, it is possible that she could end up as a defendant, much to her surprise and dismay.

I guess the point is, even when you are asked to participate in something where you think you have no involvement, please, please cooperate. I have spent more time in trying to navigate my way through setting up a meeting than I would in handling a major portion of a potential claim. We are not your enemies. We represent you. Most defense counsel have been doing this kind of work for years and years, and we genuinely have the best interests of the provider at heart. Please trust us and work with us. It will save you from being involved in a potential lawsuit.

PATIENT RIGHTS

A number of cases in the past 40 years or so have found that a physician or other healthcare provider has a duty of secrecy or loyalty to a patient in the litigation process. What does this mean?

In basic terms, it means that you should never discuss your patient with anyone representing the adverse side (the doctor being sued for example), unless you know a representative of the patient is involved. Under HIPAA, for lawyers for the doctor being sued to obtain your records, they must certify that they have given notice to the attorney for the patient that they are making this request for records.

Testifying

An important matter is your potential involvement as a witness at a trial or deposition in a case involving one of your colleagues. Please always contact your insurer when you receive a request to be a witness. I assure you that doing so will make your life less complicated and help you to avoid casting stones at a colleague when you truly do not mean to do so. Do not under any circumstances speak with or communicate with the attorney for the physician who is defending a case involving your patient without the permission of your patient, and don't ever agree to be an expert witness on the opposite side of your patient. In some states, it may not be possible for you to be an expert witness on behalf of a colleague physician in a case that involves your patient. Some courts have found that you owe an absolute duty to the patient, which cannot be overridden by your agreeing to be an expert on behalf of a defendant. This raises the issue of whether it is more important to have truth in a trial process or to protect confidentiality. During the course of a lawsuit, you may have to provide your records to the attorneys representing either the patient or a physician, and you may have to give a deposition or even trial testimony in a case. The important thing is to be extraordinarily cautious in not agreeing to be "for hire" in a case that involves your own patient. You may give testimony at a trial which is favorable to a colleague but not as a "hired expert."

The Incompetent Patient

You also need to be alert for the "incompetent patient." If you are a physician practicing in the area of psychiatry, for example, you must beware of initiating treatment with antipsychotic medications for incompetent patients without the need for "substituted judgment." Most states require that the institution or facility go to a family court and petition for a "substituted judgment plan" for an incompetent patient. This is a very cumbersome procedure, but it does protect the rights of patients and protects you.

You may initiate emergency treatment of psychiatric patients with antipsychotic medications to avoid immediate, substantial and irreversible deterioration of a serious mental illness. However, this is a strictly interpreted exception to treating without consent. In most cases with incompetent patients, including incompetent patients who need surgical procedures, you need to be extremely cautious and seek legal guidance from the legal department with which you are affiliated.

Patient Self-Determination Act and Advance Directives

The issue of patient rights has been brought to the forefront recently by legislation in a number of states, as well as at the federal level by passage of the Patient Self-Determination Act (PSDA).

The PSDA and regulations that were issued in accordance with it require that hospitals, primary care clinics, skilled nursing facilities, nursing facilities, home health agencies, and hospices maintain written policies and procedures regarding what are referred to as "advance directives." The written information to patients must put them on notice of their individual rights under the law of the state where you practice relative to their making decisions concerning medical care, which includes the right to accept or refuse care and the right to have these so-called advance directives. There should be documentation in the individual's medical record if he has signed an advance directive. You cannot make it a condition of providing care that the individual either has or doesn't have such a document. This information, in the case of a hospital, is generally given to a patient at the time of admission. Education for staff is also required.

You are not required to provide care that is in conflict with the advanced written wishes of the patient. You are not required to follow an advance directive if it is a matter of conscience for you to not implement it and the law of the state where you practice allows you to conscientiously object.

A healthcare advance directive is a document that combines a living will and a healthcare power of attorney into

one. It can include directions for organ donation and pref-
erences for treatment or nontreatment, including comfort
care or pain relief, and usually names an agent and/or an
alternative to act on behalf of the patient should she be
incompetent. In the past with an incompetent patient, it was
a bureaucratic and legal jumble to have the hospital retain
an attorney to go to court to have a guardian appointed
for the patient with authority to consent to treatment or
withhold treatment.

The patient should be encouraged to have an advance
directive. Such a document will make your life easier by
having something that clearly states with whom you are
dealing. When you have questions about the validity of a
directive, you should seek legal advice, because there might
be some minor differences in the legal requirements from
state to state. Generally speaking, however, these directives
are recognized throughout the country.

Jehovah's Witnesses

Jehovah's Witnesses have been the subject of many legal
decisions over the years in all parts of the United States.
Issues arise when either the patient is a Jehovah's Witness
and incompetent and a family member is objecting to the
use of blood products that may be necessary to save the life
of the patient or the patient is a competent patient who
objects to receiving any blood products. Be aware that some
institutions, perhaps not geographically close to you, will
provide care to Jehovah's Witnesses with the understanding
that they will not use blood products. A clinician may have
religious, moral, or ethical reservations about not doing

what is necessary to save someone's life by the use of blood products, which complicates the problem.

There have been cases where hospitals have gone to court seeking an order to compel a patient to receive blood products where, in the case of a pregnant patient for example, not doing so would place the life of the fetus at risk. In other cases, where a Jehovah's Witness is the parent of very young children, the courts have intervened and acted to protect the parent-child relationship by ordering treatment of the individual, insulating the caregivers from liability for treating without consent. There have actually been some cases where patients have filed a suit naming the institution or provider, seeking an order that they not be given blood products because they have a plan in place for other people to care for their minor children. In a couple of cases around the country, courts have acceded to the wishes of the Jehovah's Witness, knowing that the patient might die leaving minor children but recognizing their right to do so on the condition that there is a plan in place for the raising and nurturing of the children.

The pancreatitis case I mentioned earlier was one in which the husband of the Jehovah's Witness gave permission and, according to the physicians, was present when the patient herself consented and expressed a desire to live, in fact signing a note to that effect. Regrettably, because of a missing record, these two physicians had to go through the ordeal of a trial based on the patient saying that she never would have assented to this invasion of her privacy and violation of her constitutional right to practice her religion, and furthermore, that even if she had given consent, she must have been on medications that precluded her from giving a competent consent.

When you have patients whose religious or personal beliefs conflict with what you feel are your obligations as a provider, you need to have a heightened awareness of the potential for being involved in litigation. The time to consult and obtain legal advice is earlier rather than later. The transfer of a patient to a facility where those rights will be recognized will, in almost all cases, prevent you from being involved in a potential lawsuit. Likewise, going to a court of appropriate jurisdiction to seek judicial relief may result in orders for a particular kind of treatment or will at least insulate you from potential liability should treatment not be ordered.

RECOGNIZE YOUR LIMITATIONS

Know Your Area of Expertise

One of the areas where we see great potential for claims is in the field of obstetrics and gynecology. Often at the specific request of a patient, certified nurse midwives who are managing the labor and delivery delay involving an obstetrician until the absolute last moment, when the crisis has reached a stage where reasoned, calm judgment cannot be applied.

We have had cases where obstetricians have been called in for a complicated shoulder dystocia case and a child ends up with a permanent injury and disability. The obstetrician, who probably had no prior physician relationship with the patient, inevitably ends up as a defendant in a lawsuit. If an obstetrical house officer or an experienced obstetrician is called to deal with a situation of shoulder dystocia and has had no prior experience with this obstetrical emergency, she should recognize her own limitations and, if time permits, get emergency assistance. This is not always possible, but better planning can help prevent these situations. I am not attempting to tread on the relationship between nurse midwives and obstetricians, but in attempting to avoid liability, more carefully drafted protocols need to be in place and the providers need to know what the protocols say.

Likewise, if you are an obstetrician performing a laparascopic procedure and have a complication where you feel you have damaged bowel or some internal organ, you should immediately obtain consultation of general surgery, urology, or whatever specialty may be available to help. This situation is not the time to take on areas of surgery for which you may not be qualified and may not have credentialing privileges in your institution.

Another example would be if you were an emergency room physician dealing with a stroke victim in the first few hours of the onset of symptoms. Your first thought should be to involve an expert neurologist. Many, if not most, hospitals have stroke protocols, and you should follow the protocol exactly. Many hospitals without neurosurgical capability have arrangements with teaching hospitals for telemedicine evaluation of stroke victims for potential use of thrombolytics. Anything you can do to show that you have acted to obtain expert advice and consultation in the care of these types of emergencies will help protect you from potential liability.

Consultations

You would think that consultations in general pose no risk of a claim against you as the referring physician. There have actually been several cases around the country where a primary care physician was sued for negligently referring a patient for "unconventional" medical treatment without informing the patient of the known risks associated with the treatment. The ultimate decision in two appeals court cases was in favor of the physician, but I point out these situations just to alert you to exercise caution in making referrals to someone whom you know may use treatment methods that are not generally accepted. In those cases, you have a duty to make a disclosure to your patient as well.

In several analogous cases, a physician has been sued for allegedly referring patients to a physician "known to be incompetent." This may seem quite incomprehensible to you as a logical person. What happens in the real world is that the plaintiff lawyer has probably learned that the physician who actually may have been negligent either has no insurance or is underinsured, and the attorney is seeking to add any other physician who might be held liable, even if it's a stretch. A plaintiff's lawyer usually will not attempt this manuever unless the patient's injuries are significant enough to try to take on a rather unlikely theory of the case. The point is, you should periodically look over the specialty physicians to whom you make referrals, just to be certain that you haven't heard anything disparaging about them with respect to their ability. It may be that the specialist to whom you regularly send patients is still using a procedure that has been generally bypassed by other physicians in that specialty. Again, knowing that this is another nuisance in your life, it doesn't hurt to update your sense of the people to whom you make referrals.

Chapter 4

Adverse Events

I CAN'T IMAGINE THAT ANY healthcare provider will go through a career without adverse events. I remember meeting with a prominent psychiatrist who was an expert for me in a case in which we were defending another psychiatrist whose patient had committed suicide shortly after being discharged from in-hospital care. The expert for the plaintiff had written an opinion letter that the discharge was inexcusable and that something like that had never happened to him. My expert commented to me, "If he hasn't had any patients commit suicide on his watch, then he is not treating very sick patients." The point is that adverse events will indeed happen, but you can diffuse them and move forward without the events inevitably turning into legal claims.

SHOULD YOU CONTINUE TREATING THE PATIENT?

One adverse event that comes to mind is a case where I was called by a hospital because a non-English-speaking patient was being worked up for generalized abdominal pain. One of the house officers interpreted an imaging study as showing an acute abdomen, probably a bowel obstruction, and the patient was taken to surgery on an emergent basis. At surgery, no obstruction was discovered, and nothing in the abdomen matched the imaging study. It was then learned that the house officer had been looking at the imaging study of a different patient. The patient was returned to her room, having undergone an exploratory laparotomy for no reason. The next day, when she was able to transfer from the hospital bed to a chair, the food delivery service ran over her foot with the food cart, breaking her foot. That's when I received a call: "What should we do?" My first suggestion was to transfer this lady to a hotel where we couldn't do more harm to her. Hospital administrative people met with this woman and her family, apologized, and told them that they would not receive any bills for any of the hospitalization. Surprisingly, this case never turned into a lawsuit.

Another case that comes to mind was a situation where a surgeon was performing abdominal surgery on a morbidly obese woman and a towel was left in the wound. Like most hospitals, this one had a practice of counting surgical sponges but not towels. The towel had been used to hold some of the abdominal contents out of the way during the course of the surgery, and it somehow got caught up in the intestines and was not visible when the wound was closed.

The woman returned postoperatively with apparent signs of a wound infection. Imaging studies showed that some foreign object was present. The towel was not radio-opaque and did not show up clearly on a plain film. The surgeon sat with the patient and explained to her what had happened and told her that he needed to operate again, which he did. The towel was removed without any further complications. Billing was done in the usual manner. The patient thanked the surgeon profusely. Two years later, she and her husband filed a lawsuit against the surgeon and the institution, and the case ended up being settled.

How to Deal with the Patient/Family If You Continue Treatment

If, in fact, you continue to treat a patient after an adverse event, you need to be extra vigilant in your concern for the patient, spending enough time with the patient to address any and all concerns he might have. Most people under-stand that not everyone is perfect, and they will forgive you for a large number of misadventures if you handle them properly.

I mentioned earlier a situation in which a surgeon had marked an operative site but as the surgical procedure began, the operative site was obscured by the drapes. When the surgeon looked at the young patient, it appeared that the nonoperative site was more symptomatic than the one that was planned for the surgery. After the surgeon had made the initial incisions but before he began the more complex part of the procedure, the nurse anesthetist who had relieved the anesthesiologist looked at the operative permit and noted that they were doing the incorrect site. She informed the surgeon, the surgery was stopped, and the surgeon left the room to speak with the family. This openness with the family probably has averted a lawsuit, although it's still too early to tell. The surgeon told the family that he had begun a procedure on the incorrect site and made a full disclosure of the reasons why the mistake occurred. He also offered to stop the procedure as it was at the present time or, if they wished, to go forward with the planned procedure on the correct site. The family asked that he go forward with the procedure and he did.

He has had several meetings with the family since then and has continued to be the attending physician for this youngster, who had a very good result from the surgery and in the long term will probably have minimal, if any, obvious scarring from the two incisions on the incorrect side. This is another example of the correct way to deal with adverse events, showing how most patients will react to a full disclosure. Most patients are irritated and angry when they get the impression that things have been concealed from them, and these emotions are exactly what drives them to a lawyer's office. We will discuss this further, but often, full disclosure is the best preventive medicine to a potential medical malpractice claim.

As an example of proactive full disclosure, you need to be quite cautious if you are an obstetrician, or a family care physician who is doing obstetrical care, about giving patients the impression that you will be the physician present at the labor and delivery of their baby. Cases have been brought throughout the country where patients have sued their primary healthcare provider during the prenatal care for not being present at the labor and delivery, when complications occurred causing disability to the child. Never promise to be present for delivery. Even if you have a very special patient with whom you feel a close relationship, it may not always be possible or practical for you to show up at the delivery. Who knows what can intervene that would result in your not being there, and God forbid, if something adverse happens, you will be subjected to a claim. Be very careful about promising anything, particularly whether you will be physically present at anything, including a delivery.

COMMUNICATING WITH THE PATIENT/ FAMILY AFTER AN ADVERSE EVENT

When encountering an adverse event, to avoid a formal claim, you have to consider whether you wish to "apologize" to the patient. You should never ignore complaints from a patient. You should investigate the complaint, be tactful, document phone calls, and certainly determine whether you and/or your office wish to reduce or waive a particular bill. Doing so can save you a nightmare of months and months of unpleasantness involving one of these cases.

It may always be wise to obtain medical consultation, and if you sense that the family is not comfortable with you following up, to arrange for some other physician to treat the patient in the future. You should always offer to be available, and it's a very good idea to follow up with the physician to whom you may refer the patient, as well as with the patient.

Initial Patient/Family Meeting

Obviously, immediately after an adverse event, you need to speak with the patient and family members to tell them what happened and help them understand its potential consequences. You should try to answer questions directly and, always, truthfully. You should always be emotionally supportive and never blame another physician. Never speculate about what may have happened, because such speculation may prove to be inaccurate as things go forward.

Meeting with the Healthcare Team

Arrangements should be made for a meeting with the rest of the healthcare team, and having a team meeting prior to meeting with the family is highly advisable so that everyone is on the same page. You want to eliminate any potential conflicts among providers in relaying information to the patient and family. Someone should be identified as the leading voice of the providers in communicating with the patient or the patient's family after one of these events. Certainly, you should contact your organization's risk manager for advice as to how best to proceed with this entire process.

Subsequent Patient/Family Meeting(s)

After the initial, immediate meeting with the patient and family members, an additional meeting should take place with the same people to try to generate a common understanding of what might have happened, how it might have damaged the patient, the patient's outlook for the future, and what you could do to help prevent something like this from happening again. You should arrange to be available for further contacts from the patient and the patient's family, particularly as they truly begin to understand what has happened and think of new questions.

How to Apologize

Try not to be defensive; you should certainly acknowledge and even apologize for the great distress to the patient. However, you should not accept blame or even assign blame to any others, and do not criticize the care of anybody else. Apologizing is not necessarily the same as saying that you were at fault. One can express regret that something happened without shouldering blame for the event. Most states recognize that if a physician apologizes to a patient for something bad that happened, the apology is not necessarily an admission of liability and is not admissible in a subsequent malpractice case as an admission of liability. You should always be willing to speak with patients and their families regarding errors and to apologize and express deep sympathy. Doing so can go a long way to lowering the temperature in a situation where people are thinking of litigation. Remember, too, that you never know what member of a family, aside from the patient, will trigger a claim.

What do you do about apologizing to patients and patients' families when something really bad happens in the course of the care and treatment of a patient? Linda Crawford, who teaches trial advocacy at Harvard Law School and consults with defendants on research-based effectiveness in medical malpractice cases, and whom I consider to be a friend, has helped us and has also written extensively about these situations. She has written articles about whether or not apologies help to reduce litigation, and she, along with many others, have wondered about the validity of an apology program in the medical practice setting. Some hospitals in our area with which I am familiar take affirmative approaches to meeting immediately with families when something bad happens and being quite forthright.

One of the obstacles to having a legitimate apology program is that it may include some compensation in dollars to the patient. Providers have become quite creative in fashioning remedies such as waiving bills, creating new programs in the name of the patient or outright memorials, which need no reporting. If indeed compensation is paid to the patient, this becomes a reportable event to the National Practitioner Data Bank. Reportability is really what makes it difficult for physicians and other healthcare providers to acknowledge mistakes and to engage in reconciliation with the patient and/or the patient's family. It has been shown that an apology program can reduce litigation and perhaps the cost of medical malpractice claims. Until some progress is made in modifying the reporting situation with the National Practitioner Data Bank, however, such programs will not make much progress. Some of these situations are handled more easily in governmental hospitals, such as those of the U.S. Department of Veterans Affairs, where employed physicians have no personal liability and a payment made to a patient or a patient's family is not necessarily a reportable event.

While major events will still most likely precipitate lawsuits, programs that facilitate early meetings with families and patients certainly would help in eliminating the relatively minor claims from less severe injuries. As Linda Crawford has written, the severity of the injury seems to matter the most, so it is not clear whether the apology situation will help to eliminate malpractice claims when a patient suffers very serious injuries or other consequences. This area is still being studied, but it has the potential to be of assistance to physicians and insurers in reducing the overall number of claims.

The Role of Risk Management and the Insurance Carrier

If the event occurred in the inpatient setting, you should contact the appropriate risk manager, both for notification purposes and to seek that person's assistance. Also, you should not be reluctant to notify your malpractice insurance carrier. As a clinician, you will not be penalized for telling the carrier about a possible claim. Most insurers do not make a true claim record until they formally receive a claim or a lawsuit. Potential claims should not be used to calculate your premiums, but they may be useful in identifying potential quality of care issues or defective equipment that requires notification to a manufacturer or a supplier.

Responding to a Written Complaint

If you have a written complaint from a patient or a family member and you suspect that it may turn into a formal claim, you should very quickly respond by letting the person know that you will collect information, attempt to solve whatever problem he has raised, and will get back to him quickly. That last step is the most important one: you need to get back to the individual as quickly as possible. Sometimes ignoring even a relatively minor complaint can lead to a lawsuit. You should investigate what happened, read the record, and, if applicable, speak with other providers who may have been present or involved in the care of a patient. When you feel comfortable that you have all of the facts, you should either respond in writing, with the assistance of your risk manager or a representative of your insurer, or meet with the people in person. If you have an in-person meeting, I recommend that a staff member in your office be present, because there is always the opportunity for miscommunication.

As mentioned in chapter 3 in the section "Hospital Records," a case arose involving a difficult delivery involving shoulder dystocia in which the defendants, particularly the nurse midwife, were alleged to have used excessive force, resulting in fracturing the neck of the fetus and causing its death. The parents of this baby were non-English speaking. After the incident, they met with patient representatives from the hospital and some members of the treatment team, who were called away frequently, disrupting the meeting. Also, the translator did not accurately grasp the medical situation as it was explained. Although X-rays revealed no fracture, they did show some soft tissue injury to the neck; as this finding was communicated and translated at a later meeting, the parents got the definite impression that "the baby's neck had been broken." As I mentioned previously, systemic problems resulting in "missing" X-rays complicated the defense.

The legal consequences arising from this terribly sad event might have been avoided by taking the following steps:

- Installing a procedure or contractual requirement whereby the referring hospital, which paid for the autopsy, required the hospital where the autopsy was being performed to return to it any X-rays or lab work done. These results could then be kept with the mother's record for future reference.
- Handling the family meetings better. If there had been better communication among the parties with the aid of competent translators, the whole legal event might have been averted.

Dealing with the Bill

Whether you should reduce or even waive a bill is ultimately up to you and/or your practice, but you need to make sure it does not come across as an admission of fault or liability. It can be offered as a gesture of goodwill to the patient or the patient's family: simply tell them that you are sorry that they had this complication or unexpected event, you appreciate the physician-patient relationship you have with them, and you have asked your billing office to delete all or part of the bill. The important thing is to see to it that this is carried out. The worst scenario would be if somehow the bill ends up at a collection agency and the patient receives dunning letters. This is a sure precipitant of a trip to a lawyer. Experience has shown that in many cases when a bill is reduced with appropriate compassion for the patient, that patient never pursues a malpractice claim. Other people may pursue the malpractice claim whether you write off the bill or not. In such cases, an adjustment to a bill should not be considered an admission of liability, although it will call for explanation should the case actually end up in a courtroom.

Record Keeping

Obviously, as soon as possible after an adverse event occurs, you need to record what happened and how you responded. Never alter anything and never back-date any information. You should not write anything in the medical record with respect to notifying risk management, a legal department, or your insurer or even that an incident report was filed. Such information is not part of the treatment record of the patient and only serves as a red flag for a plaintiff and/or her legal representative who reviews the records later.

Whatever steps can be taken to preserve the record and/or evidence of what occurred should be taken. For years, I have told people at meetings not to return devices to the manufacturer when they feel a mishap was contributed to or directly caused by the device. I can almost guarantee that you will never see that device again and, thus, will never be able to test it. Device malfunctions are better left in the hands of the risk management people at your facility. Sometimes it's appropriate to have photographs taken as soon as possible, particularly if a slip-and-fall or a wall-hanging device may have malfunctioned, so that some evidence is preserved of what occurred as soon as possible after the event.

Recap: Procedures to Follow

Remember that early compassion for the patient and the family may be the key to preventing rather than escalating a situation. Always be positive and never blame yourself or anyone else for what may have happened. It would be wise to do the following:

- Where appropriate, obtain consultation and, in some cases, consultation outside the hospital or other setting where the event occurred.
- Contact the risk manager and/or your malpractice insurer.
- Make arrangements to follow up with the patient.
- Be sure that someone will be available to coordinate the response to the family.
- Speak with the team members about what happened and make sure that you have straightened out any disagreements as to what happened before meeting with the patient or family.
- Have a family meeting with you and other members of the team if applicable, with a

staff member available to sit in on the entire
meeting.

- Tell the family that you are absolutely available
  for follow-up of a solution to any complaint
  they have and to listen to any further complaints surrounding their care. This is not
  the time to accept "blame" or to criticize anyone else.
- Be available for repeated conversations with
  the patient.
- If a medical device was involved and there is
  a question of whether that device performed
  adequately, this is a good reason to involve
  professionals who can arrange appropriate
  testing of the device.
- In the case of medical device problems, there
  may be reporting requirements, or it may
  simply be wise to report the incident to appropriate governmental agencies.

Managing the physician-patient relationship to avoid
a claim after an adverse event requires compassion, communication, and a great deal of time but may prove extraordinarily beneficial for everyone involved. So many times
we have had people say, "The doctor never told me what
went wrong," "No one told me what really happened," or "I
never really understood what happened in the course of my
treatment or my relative's treatment until I heard it here in
a courtroom." This is not a good way to practice medicine,
such that a patient only fully understands what happened

upon hearing testimony in a trial. You need to avoid the process altogether.

WHAT HAPPENS IF YOU ARE SUED?

Despite your best efforts, someone has made a claim against you, whether it be by a claim letter, a telephone call, or a formal summons and/or complaint. What do you do now? First of all, *never* communicate directly with the patient or the patient's attorney after you receive notice of a formal claim. You should immediately report this claim to your insurer, your risk manager, and/or your office practice manager and sit back and wait for them to help you.

Did I mention *never* to communicate with your patient or the patient's attorney? This is now a highly adversarial relationship, and you need to be alert to the best possible ways to protect your own interests. Many physicians feel that they can contact a patient and convince him that the course of treatment was well within the standard of care and that they have done nothing wrong. All this does is give rise to a situation where you have made a potential admission of liability, which will be grossly detrimental down the road.

Again, I cannot emphasize enough that you should *not* communicate with anyone other than people who are acting in your behalf and with your best interest at heart. Depending on whether you have received a preliminary claim letter or a formal summons and complaint, you still will need to develop relationships among you, your insurer, and an attorney who will be appointed to represent your best interests.

Another point to keep in mind: Do not transfer personal property out of your name. For example, if you transferred the title of your personal residence solely to your spouse or to a family trust immediately after notification of a potential claim, this action could be construed as an admission of liability. You would look as though you were trying to hide assets from a potential judgment. You may still conduct "arms-length" transactions after a claim is filed. In other words, you would be perfectly justified in participating in a legitimate sale of your property or purchase of another property, as long as it is truly an "arms-length" transaction; that is, one resulting from the customary relationship in the marketplace of a seller and buyer.

Insurer-Attorney Relationship

The legal relationship between your attorney and you is similar to your relationship with a patient and the patient's health insurer. While your attorney may be paid by your medical malpractice insurer, the primary responsibility of that lawyer is to you with a secondary responsibility to the insurer. In almost every state of which I am aware, this is the case. Again, it is the primary responsibility of your lawyer to act in your best interest. I really believe that you will find that medical malpractice insurers historically have acted in the best interest of insured physicians in processing medical malpractice claims.

How Does a Suit Begin?

Following are some preliminary steps of which you should be aware.

The Formal Complaint. A claim is generally begun by the filing of a complaint by the plaintiff in a court, as well as service upon you, either formally by sheriff's or constable's representative or by acceptance of service of process by your attorney or insurer. The formal complaint is generally written in the broadest of terms and doesn't really tell you a great deal about the nature of the case. Sometimes it contains quite inflammatory allegations, which you should not be terribly concerned about. We see these all the time. No matter what is alleged, don't take these allegations to heart, as many of them are formalistic and appear in every case that a particular plaintiff may file. The answer, equally nonspecific and pro forma, consists primarily of a denial of 99 percent of the allegations set forth by the plaintiff. Only as things play out will you be able to detect the true nature of the complaint of the patient and the true medical-legal basis for the allegations.

We generally request preliminary hearings to see if the case has sufficient merit to go forward without requiring the plaintiff to initiate pretrial bonding or some other appropriate procedure, depending on the state in which you live.

Meeting with the Claim Representative. Early in the process, you will be asked to meet with a claim representative of your insurer and/or the law firm selected to represent you. You need to be prepared for this meeting and to set aside sufficient time in your schedule for it. After all, this person is there to represent you and your interests. It is understandable that you would think that these meetings need to be conducted outside of your normal schedule, but you need to bear in mind that claims representatives and attorneys are busy professionals who also have lives to lead; you can't expect that they will meet with you at abnormal hours. Remember that they are not being sued and that they are appointed and acting on your behalf. Please try to be cooperative with them. Before meeting with your legal representatives and insurer representatives, you should make certain that they have a full and complete copy of the medical record in question and that you have reviewed the record yourself. Preparation will expedite the process and be productive and beneficial to your defense.

Screening the Claim. After the initial filing of the complaint, the plaintiff or patient's attorney must undergo the process of screening the claim through a so-called medical malpractice tribunal or will have to get a preliminary expert opinion, which they file with the complaint. These requirements vary from state to state, so you need to check with your particular jurisdiction. However, all states have the same essential requirements in common: the plaintiff needs to show to a court that she has sufficient basis for bringing a potential medical malpractice case and going forward with it.

In states that provide for medical malpractice tribunal screening, at some point a tribunal will be convened, which may consist of a judge alone or, in some states, a judge with a medical member from your specialty and an attorney member. The tribunal will hold a rather cursory hearing into whether the plaintiff has sufficient basis for the claim to proceed. In most instances, when the plaintiff has an expert opinion from almost any physician, in any specialty, he will be allowed to proceed toward trial.

In the event that plaintiffs are unsuccessful at the tribunal stage, they generally are required to furnish a bond in some amount to pursue the case. Most plaintiff lawyers who feel that they have a legitimate case are well prepared to deal with this contingency. If they have a medical malpractice tribunal hearing and are ordered to post a bond to avoid dismissal of the case, they will post the bond and proceed to trial.

One of the advantages of the tribunal process in most states is that it gives the defense an early opportunity to get a better idea of the true basis of the complaint. The experts produced at the tribunal, by written report, are not necessarily the same experts who will show up at trial. We do, however, have an early opportunity to see a more definite and, hopefully, scientific explanation of the theory of the plaintiff's case.

The Emotional Burden. It is certainly unsettling to anyone to have a deputy sheriff or process server show up at one's office or home with a complaint and summons containing, in the vaguest of terms, remarkable and greatly exaggerated allegations of wrongdoing. Again, bear in mind that these complaints are generally "one size fits all." Try not to take it terribly to heart.

Although I am unaware of any documented clinical studies, there is certainly significant emotional trauma to a provider and the provider's family in a malpractice suit. The most appropriate way to respond to the initial bad news is to contact your insurer immediately. Your insurer will then assign a claim representative to the case and will make arrangements for the appointment of an attorney to represent your interests. Attorneys who do medical defense work are generally well-seasoned specialists in medical-legal situations. I'll say it again: you should never, under any circumstances, attempt to contact the patient or the lawyer who has brought the claim against you. Doing so will return to haunt you during the course of litigation.

You should not feel that you are an inferior physician merely because allegations have been made. The vast majority of medical malpractice cases that are tried to conclusion are resolved in favor of the physician.

Physician support groups around the country help providers who are having difficulty coping with the litigation process. You should take advantage of these resources when necessary. Often, malpractice insurance companies provide psychological counseling, which is completely private and confidential and can be of assistance to get you through any emotional turmoil you experience.

How Does a Suit Go Forward?

Discovery. After this initial foray, the parties generally engage in written and oral discovery.

The parties on both sides send rather formal written questions, or *interrogatories,* to each other. You will be sent those questions by your attorney with some suggestions and/or assistance as to how you should respond. These are formal court proceedings, and they need to be responded to in a timely fashion.

Ordinarily, after the written discovery period, the parties engage in something called *depositions,* although different terms are used in different states. You are usually required to appear at the office of the opposing attorney to give oral testimony. If location, location, location is the secret to selling real estate, then preparation, preparation, preparation is the key to success in a deposition. Your attorney will meet with you beforehand to help prepare you for your deposition. Depositions can be a significant part of any medical malpractice case, and I urge you to be prepared and to cooperate with your lawyer, who has done this many times. We can only do so much unless you participate in the process. The actual deposition will be before a court reporter, and you will be required to testify under oath. Sometimes, depending on the state in which the case is filed, the deposition may be videotaped.

In most cases, your own attorney will not ask questions at such a proceeding, because it is meant to aid the discovery only of the opposing party. At deposition, the general rule is "don't volunteer too much information." You are there only to answer the questions of the opposing party and not necessarily to disclose every tidbit of information about your care and treatment of the patient. This information about your care will come out at the time of trial. You need to resist the temptation to be a "teacher" or a "volunteer of information." Just answer the questions that are put to you by the lawyer at your discovery deposition. Your legal team, at an appropriate time, such as at trial, will extract the full story from you with questions that will give you an opportunity to tell your side of the matter.

Don't talk too much at your deposition. I am reminded of an old friend of mine who was the chief of orthopedics at a large Boston area hospital. He and I had done a number of educational programs for physicians in the medical-legal area. I referred to him as being an advocate of the "Calvin Coolidge College of Testifying." His theory was, after reviewing many deposition transcripts of doctors, that doctors talk too much and get themselves in trouble during the deposition process. He felt that the defendant doctors should answer questions with one word, in some situations with two words, but rarely with three or more words. His advice would be, if you found yourself speaking in complete sentences, to stop and ask the lawyer to repeat the question. He was always a big hit with the medical audience. I think that his approach is a bit too extreme, but it makes the point well that you should be brief and just respond to the questions. You may be feeling an irresistible impulse to elaborate on some point that you think will be extraordinarily helpful to your case and feel frustrated that the opponent doesn't ask you the key question. Don't volunteer the information.

Expert Review. As the case goes forward, your insurer, with the cooperation of and input from your attorney, will have the case reviewed by experts in your field and, in many situations, by experts who have particular skill and knowledge in areas such as causation to determine if you have complied with the standard of care and whether or not any compliance or failure to comply with the standard of care may have contributed to causing injury or death.

You should understand that we are highly reluctant to tell you if we have had expert reviews by individuals who may be critical of your care and treatment. These people would never be willing to do expert reviews again if they knew we were going to tell our clients that they had criticized their role in the care of a patient. We will tell you the general nature of any criticism, and, obviously, when we know that we have experts who are available to be witnesses at trial, we will fully identify those people. It is most awkward to be in a situation where a client of ours knows that we have a potential expert who is not supportive and it happens to be someone with whom they have a slight professional relationship. Please trust the process to your attorney and/or insurance claim representative so that we can act as objectively as possible in your behalf.

By the way, without ready, willing, and able experts, it would be impossible for us to try these cases successfully. If you have ever been asked to be an expert in the past and declined, I would recommend that you rethink that position and agree to be part of the adjudicatory process as an expert in the future.

Disposal of the Case

For many years, I have told new clients that cases are disposed of in only three ways:

1. Voluntary dismissal by the plaintiff or patient
2. Settlement
3. Trial

Each of these potential outcomes has subcategories.

Dismissal. In the subcategory of dismissal, sometimes there are legal grounds to file certain motions to dismiss a case. Perhaps the plaintiff failed to bring the claim within the statutorily required time limit (the statute of limitations). Other legal bases exist as well for motions to have a case dismissed. Also, sometimes during the course of discovery, the plaintiff feels that she either does not have valid grounds to go forward or the client does not want the expense of pursing a case for years to a conclusion by a trial, and she voluntarily entertains dismissal.

Settlement. After the claim has been reviewed by experts retained by your insurer or attorney, it may be apparent that the case will be very difficult to defend at trial. In these circumstances, with your knowledge, and in some states, your prior approval, negotiations will take place to effect a settlement. We often engage the services of an independent mediator to facilitate the process. We also make all efforts to maintain confidentiality of the settlement, other than required reporting.

Trial. Under the category of trial, the case could be heard by a fact finder other than a traditional jury. It has become much more common to have cases adjudicated by arbitrators. Arbitrators are generally people whom both sides agree on to dispose of the case. They often are retired judges or people in whom both parties have a good deal of confidence to pass upon a case in a binding fashion. Arbitrators are not to be confused with mediators, with whom I will deal in a few moments. Healthcare providers are usually much more comfortable submitting a case to binding arbitration than putting it before a jury. Instead of a lengthy two- or three-week trial, an arbitrated case may involve one, two, or three days in a private setting and result in a binding decision one way or the other. To submit to arbitration does not mean that a case cannot be determined in favor of the healthcare provider. Arbitration has all of the consequences of a full hearing, just without the 12-, 14-, or whatever-member jury your state requires.

Arbitration is generally agreed upon by the parties to be "final." The findings of the arbitrator are absolutely final, and you will not be involved in any lengthy appeals process, which can often be the case in a jury trial. The downside is that if you lose at arbitration, that is also a final, binding decision.

Mediation, on the other hand, is a process whereby the parties agree to meet with an impartial individual who attempts to "mediate" the differences between the parties. In a medical malpractice case, mediation is generally used in situations where your insurer and you have agreed that the case should be settled but the parties are not in agreement as to the financial terms. It is not productive to go to mediation if you are not agreeable to an actual settlement. In the past, we always informed doctors that a "settlement" was a reasonable disposition to a number of cases. Today with the reporting requirements to the National Practitioner Data Bank, you need to be aware that any negotiated settlement will be reported to the Data Bank and you will be questioned with respect to it for ten years. You should also be aware that many physicians have settled cases without any impact on their clinical privileges or rights to practice medicine, and having settled a case is not a particular "black mark" on you or your clinical skills. In many cases, you may have supportive expert reviews, but a settlement is made anyway on the basis of pure economic reality, knowing that the potential verdict for a plaintiff could be astronomic and damaging to you personally and financially. The consequences need to be weighed by you, your family, and your personal attorney before entering into mediation.

Cooperate with Your Attorney

Your cooperation is an essential part of the ease with which you will pass through the litigation process. It is most frustrating to a defense attorney to have an uncooperative provider as a client. We can only do our best and obtain the best results for you when we have your complete and full cooperation. That means that you may have to interrupt your busy schedule to accommodate your attorney, who will, I assure you, do his best to disrupt your regular professional routine as little as possible. You must learn to trust your defense lawyer, much as you would expect a patient to experience the relationship with you as a physician. If that can be accomplished and you have a good relationship with your defense attorney, then the whole process will be less traumatic.

Frequently, defense lawyers will advise you not to discuss the case with any other treating physicians without the approval of your defense team. You will be asked later, either in written discovery, oral depositions, or at trial, whether you spoke with any other physicians regarding the case. When this happens during discovery, I assure you that a careful plaintiff lawyer will seek to take the deposition of the individual with whom you spoke. This can complicate your defense and inconveniences individuals who are not involved in the situation that gave rise to the case. After you have been deposed, it would be permissible for you to talk with other providers, again with approval of your defense team, but don't do so in the early stages of the claim.

You should meet with your defense team as early in the process as possible. This may mean setting aside sufficient time, without interruption, for you and them to make the most of that session. Very often, defense lawyers will go to the physician's office, at least for the initial meeting. Please try to accommodate them at reasonable times, which may mean that you do not see a full complement of patients some days. It is very frustrating to travel some distance to a physician's office for a 4:00 PM or 5:00 PM appointment and be told that the doctor will still be seeing patients for another hour or so. That's not a good way to start off the attorney-client relationship. Bear in mind that you are now a defendant in a case, and we are there to try to help you. We do know how busy you are, but it is not always possible for us to meet with our own clients in the evening. We have family obligations as well, and we spend a great deal of time outside of regular business hours meeting with experts. The experts in the medical negligence cases are not defendants in a case, and we need to accommodate them. Please be understanding of the fact that we have demands on our time as well; if you do so, you can be sure to have a good working relationship with your legal team.

It is generally good practice for the defense attorney to keep you posted of developments as the case goes forward. Some lawyers may send too much information to you so that every time you see an envelope with the name of the firm on it, it brings back the memory of the pending legal case. You should keep a file apart from the patient file for legal correspondence.

Bear in mind that you are our first line of defense, and we may need your expert input as we go forward. Make yourself available and respond when requested. Sometimes we have court deadlines with which we must comply, and we need you to review things before presenting them to a judge. I hate to tell you how many times that we have written repeatedly to a physician client with no response. It has gotten better with the use of email, because most physicians tend to review and respond personally to their email.

Please answer our letters and calls so that we can have a mutually beneficial and trusting relationship. If for some reason you are unhappy, for good reason, with your defense counsel, you can discuss that with your insurer and request someone else. You obviously have a right to involve your personal attorney in the case, but I can assure you that the people who do medical defense work are true specialists in the field. You obviously would need to pay personally for the services of your private attorney, but if you do so, we are generally happy to keep her in the loop and inform her of things as we go forward. Often, when we think it appropriate for you to consult with your own attorney, we suggest that you do so.

One of the most common complaints that I have had and that I hear from my colleagues is that in attempting to contact a client, we frequently can't get by members of your staff who are quite skillful in protecting you from outside interference. We try not to disclose that we are acting as your attorney in any particular matter; when we make a call, we say that it is a personal call and ask if the physician could return it. We are met with questions—What is your birth date? What is the problem that you wanted to discuss with the doctor?—so it is advisable to establish a procedure right at the outset. There should be a contact person in your office who knows who the people are who will be working in your defense. If you have a private line or cell phone where we can reach you directly, that is also most useful. You should tell us at the beginning whether you wish us to communicate with you in writing to your home or your office address and what would be the least intrusive or embarrassing way for us to call. We certainly would never call and tell someone in your office that we are your lawyer in a medical malpractice case. Help us establish a workable process.

When selecting experts to review the case that has now been filed against you, we and your insurer will look to people with expertise in your specialty and in the condition or problem of which a plaintiff/patient is complaining. We do literature searches to come up with the current medical literature, but in this area, you can be helpful as well. If you are aware of sources in the literature, you should let your attorney know. Don't do this without talking with your attorney, as the plaintiff lawyer will ask you at your deposition if you did a literature review and if you have kept any articles. You may have unearthed some articles that are not completely supportive of what you did, or your literature search may reveal some articles that support what you did and some that are critical of what you did. If these articles are generated by your defense, or at least at your lawyer's request, they would be protected by the attorney-client privilege and not generally discoverable by the opposite side.

You may suggest people to serve as experts, but you need to bear in mind that we need to deal with experts who will not only be willing to review the case but will be willing to appear personally in court should the case go to trial. It does us no good to have the world's leading expert review the case if we can't get him to come from another part of the country on relatively short notice to appear in court.

As discussed above, the expert or experts should never be individuals who have a personal acquaintance with you, as the relationship obviously would color their reviews. When we have unfavorable expert reviews, we generally will not tell you the name of the individual who did the review. While we will provide you with copies of the supportive reviews when we identify the experts who will appear in court on your behalf, these are materials that you should not review prior to your oral deposition because of the potential discoverability by the plaintiff.

Jurors like to hear from experts, but they really want to hear from you. What were your reasons for a particular decision and/or a particular course of treatment? It is essential for a jury to like you and to be left with the feeling that you are a caring, concerned physician. Follow your attorney's advice with respect to whether your spouse should be present for all, or a portion, of the trial. Depending on the nature of the case, I generally advise physicians not to have a spouse present, as I have seen spouses get too wrapped up in the case and end up getting into heated discussions with people from the other side. In rare cases, members of the press were involved. On a case-by-case basis, if it will not make you more nervous, spousal presence can be helpful. Consult your attorney also regarding how you should dress, both for the deposition and at the trial.

Example: The Stylish Pediatrician. One of my partners was defending a pediatrician who was being sued because he did not come to the hospital for a delivery. He had met with the young couple and agreed to be the pediatrician when the mother delivered her baby. When he received the call from the hospital, he asked or was informed that the gestational age in this case was only 19 weeks. He felt that this was clearly not a viable infant, and he chose not to show up. The parents were offended because this infant had some breathing. Most likely, the "breathing" was agonal respirations, but to them it appeared that their infant had been born alive and would have had some chance of survival if the doctor had showed up. Obviously, the whole incident could have been prevented by the doctor's going to the hospital or at least speaking with the people involved.

In any event, when the doctor came to have a full-day preparation session with my partner, I was asked to play the part of the plaintiff's lawyer. When I walked into the room,

I immediately noticed that the doctor was not dressed like the usual pediatrician whom I have seen in my experience. Most pediatricians, at least the men, wear khaki pants, casual shoes, and some type of child-friendly UNESCO necktie. This gentleman was dressed like a lawyer on his way to argue a case in the Supreme Court. I told him, "I don't like your suit." That got us started on the right footing! When we finished for the day, I told him that I thought that he was a terrific dresser but that he didn't look the part of a pediatrician. I suggested that if he had a blue blazer and/or a tweed sport jacket, that should be his uniform for the trial. I must say that he was very compliant, and my partner informed me that he alternated between a blue blazer and a sport coat for a three-week trial, which happily ended with a finding in his favor.

These may seem like small things, but they're important. It's also important for you to look at jurors when you are talking with them, to speak in a conversational tone, and to be able to explain complicated medicine at a level where each and every juror of varying education will be able to understand what you are saying in your defense.

Unlike medicine, where scientific breakthroughs occur rapidly, the legal process moves at the speed of a tortoise. You need to be prepared for a lengthy process, except in the relatively rare situation where a court accelerates the process, sometimes due to the soon expected death of a plaintiff. You will not always get adequate notice of when you have to appear, particularly at trial. These cases are frequently continued because of unavailability of one or more of the lawyers or one or more of the expert witnesses who are scheduled to testify and, obviously, when the court is unable to reach the case because of some other engagement. Providers have a great deal of difficulty in coping with the looser and somewhat inadequate legal scheduling of the process. People I talk with, such as emergency physicians or radiologists, know what their schedule is six or eight months, or even more, in advance. We tell them not to block out time for a potential trial so far in advance, because our system doesn't work as well. Please try to understand the vagaries of scheduling from our side. We truly do our best to intrude as little as possible upon your professional and personal life.

As the case slowly inches its way toward a conclusion, whether it be by dismissal, settlement, or trial, you should have a grasp of what the theory of liability is of the plaintiff and, conversely, what the theory of the defense is from a medical standpoint. Pay careful attention to the process so that you feel reasonably comfortable with the medical theory that is going to be your defense as elucidated by you and experts on your behalf. You and your experts need to be on the same page in order to have a solid, substantial, and successful defense. I have had clients call me a day or two before the start of a trial to tell me that they had a completely different theory for the defense of the case and that we needed to obtain a continuance so that we could develop that new theory. These kinds of things never sit well with any judge who is trying his best to sort out his many cases and keep them reasonably on track.

I once had an expert witness in a lithium toxicity case who showed up the day of the trial and, much to my surprise, said, "I don't think that this is really lithium toxicity."

This was a complete departure from everything that he had told us in the expert meetings and office meetings with the expert to prepare for trial. Not a good way to start a trial!

Trial by Jury

Let's assume that the case is headed for disposition by jury trial. The number of jurors may vary from 6 to, more commonly, 12 or, if the case is expected to be lengthy, even more. You need to plan to be present throughout the trial. Any exceptions to this general rule must be gone over carefully with your defense team. Jurors do not look favorably on a physician who doesn't feel the case is important enough to demand her personal attendance.

The process of selecting jurors can be laborious, and you will probably never be satisfied that you have a jury of your "peers." When you see the jurors seated in the jury box, you will probably wonder how they can ever sort through some quite complicated medical and scientific data. I have been amazed over the years at how collectively intelligent juries are. We have talked with jurors after trials, and we have conducted focus groups and mock trials. Remarkably, some one or two jurors will get a particular point and then explain it to the other jurors, and others will latch on to another particular point and explain it, and when they deliberate about the case, they generally have a quite reasonable grasp of what happened. It is not a very scientific process, but it is the best process that we have developed in our democratic form of government.

The jury is now seated, and for the first time in a public setting, you will be subjected to verbal allegations by the attorney for the patient that will elicit emotions ranging from embarrassment to blood-boiling rage. You must be stoic! This is one of the reasons why we do not like to have family members at portions of a trial, because they have a hard time acting indifferent toward allegations that may be totally unfounded and being directed at a loved one. Some plaintiff attorneys engage in really personal attacks on you, including finger pointing and other obnoxious behavior—hopefully a reasonable trial judge limits this. The good news is that within seconds of the completion of the plaintiff's opening statement, your lawyer has an opportunity to introduce you to the jury and to tell them your side of the situation. Most people are very understanding of the fact that there are at least two sides to every story and that a malpractice case is no different.

The actual trial then proceeds with what is generally a very sad and sympathetic story of what may have happened to the patient/plaintiff. You really don't have much sympathy on your side as a physician, unless jurors can relate to the fact that they could be the subject of a lawsuit or a claim for whatever it is they do for a living. I have found over the years that juries, while sympathetic to these cases, are often remarkably able to put their emotions aside and decide the case on the facts.

Perhaps the hardest part of the case for you will be listening to experts for the plaintiff criticize your treatment and say that it was way below the standard of care, perhaps even that it amounted to "gross negligence." Again, remain poker-faced and wait for your attorney to cross-examine these plaintiff's experts. Often, they are people who come with a long track record of having testified all over the country for large compensation. When this is brought out, their credibility is diminished. Sometimes they say things in the course of a trial that you would never, ever hear at a professional meeting; in fact, you would probably walk out of a meeting if a physician espoused such theories. The back-and-forth process continues with experts for the plaintiff, followed by perhaps economists and other witnesses with respect to damages, including family members and, in the very sad cases, the plaintiff will at the very end bring the damaged child to court.

At some point, the plaintiff will rest her case, and the defense has the opportunity to go forward in your behalf. However, in some cases, depending on the strategy of the plaintiff attorney, she may call you as a witness as part of their case. You need to be aware that you may be called by the opposing party before your lawyer has the opportunity to go through the details of the case with you. Generally when that happens, again depending on what state you are in, the defense attorney will reserve the right to call you later in the case as part of the defense. It is helpful that you be heard toward the latter part of the case so that the jury's memory of your testimony will be fresher when they go for deliberations. For the first time in the case, a jury will hear that you have a very good educational background and experience, that you have a family and responsibilities of your own, and that you are a caring physician. You must prepare very carefully with your lawyer for the process of testifying at trial. The impression that you leave with the jury will go a long way toward a winning result.

Now the evidence in the case has all been presented. It may be after a few days of trial, a few weeks of trial, or even a few months of trial. The general procedure is that the lawyer for the provider or defense argues first to the jury, usually for about 20 to 30 minutes, and then the lawyer for the plaintiff presents a closing argument. This is the last time you need to remain stone faced and as calm as possible during sometimes vitriolic arguments.

When the arguments are concluded, they are ordinarily followed by the judge's instructing the jury as to the law applicable to a medical malpractice case, which the jury is bound to follow in their deliberations. The case, together with all of the exhibits that may have been marked during the trial, is then sent to the jury. They retire to a secluded area to begin their deliberations.

It could be minutes, hours, or days before they return. When they do return, it is a highly emotionally charged moment when a judge or a clerk addresses the foreperson of the jury and asks, "Have the members of the jury agreed upon a verdict?" and the foreperson replies, "Yes, we have."

The ordeal is now over.

Chapter 5

Conclusion

I F I HAD TO emphasize the most important advice I could give to help you avoid a malpractice case, it would be as follows:

- Communicate with your patients so that you both have a clear understanding of your respective roles in their care.

- Communicate fully and often with colleagues of all levels so there is no misunderstanding of treatment plans for a patient.
- Know your limitations and when to call for help.
- Spend time with patients to foster the best possible patient-physician relationship.
- Update your practice with electronic records or, at a minimum, rigid safety protocols.
- Be friendly, open, and collegial with others.
- Maintain your skills by continuing education.
- When bad things happen, deal with them in a forthright manner and with the utmost compassion for your patient.
- Write letters to patients and other providers.
- Keep meticulous records.

I have the greatest admiration and affection for each and every one of you.

Acknowledgements

I WISH TO THANK MR. Josh Martino, who was the Editor at Kaplan who had the idea for the book, and through his Tuft University classmate, my son Philip, contacted me to see if I knew anyone who might be interested. And here I am.

Thanks to my wife, Christel, for putting up with me through the process.

I would also like to thank Ms. Margena Johnson for putting up with me through many revisions of 250 pages or so of manuscript, and also Sandra Degni who had to put together the first 50 pages or so.

Kudos to Michael Sprague and Dominique Polfliet at Kaplan for their editorial comments, suggestions and assistance throughout.

Index

of equipment malfunction,
146–47
by hospital staff, 104–9
misfiling of, 31
of noncompliant patient, 47–49
of telephone advice, 24–27
of treatment outside normal
standard of care, 98
of warnings given to patient, 7
Drug interactions, flagged in
electronic records, 36
Duty to warn, 5–8

E
Education, continuing, 15
"Electronic Health Records and
Malpractice Claims in Office
Practice," 38
Electronic records, 15, 35–41
advantages of, 36–39
avoiding malpractice cases with,
200
disadvantages of, 39–41
ensuring accuracy of, 39
in hospital settings, 34
pagination issues, 40
security/confidentiality and, 38
as solution to legibility problems,
130
Electronic scheduling, 21
Email communication
advice given via, 29
recordkeeping and, 24–27
Empathy, 21
Employees
cooperation of, with defense
team, 189
training office staff, 27–28
Equipment malfunction, 146,
172–73, 174
Errors
apologizing for, 167
types of, 88–92
Ethics, required reporting and, 68
"Etiquette-Based Medicine"
(Kahn), 20
Evidence-based medicine, and
guidelines, 95
Expertise, working within your area
of, 157–59

Expert reports, 10, 190
Expert review, 182–83
Expert testimony, 9, 10
requests for, 43–44, 183
selecting experts for defense, 189
Eye contact, 21

F
Fact finder, 9–10
Falls, in hospitals, 92
Family of patient, in aftermath of
adverse event, 163–65
Federal Tort Claims Act (FTCA),
79
Fetal heart tracings, 118–20
"Finding a Cure: The Case for
Regulation and Oversight
of Electronic Health Record
Systems" (Hoffman and
Podgurski), 38
Florida, practice guidelines and,
100
Foreign objects (left in patient
after surgery), 11
Formal complaint
communication following, 175,
180
filing of, 177
screening, 178–79
For-profit hospitals, 78, 81

G
Gawande, Atul, 89
Government hospitals, 78, 79
Group visits, 115–17
Guarantees, avoiding, 55
Guidelines. *See* Practice guidelines/
pathways

H
Handicapped persons, informed
consent and, 59
Handwritten notes, legibility of,
32–34, 130
Harvard Public Health Review
on checklists to avoid mistakes,
89
on electronic records, 36
Harvard Vanguard Medical
Associates, 115